MORE ADVANCE PRAISE FOR *MY MOTHER'S HOUSE*

***"Perfectly captures the personalities involved** through their humor, love, courage, and the anguish of fighting a medical system that, even if you have insurance, often does more harm than good... You're right there with the author as she seeks emotional and spiritual 'transcendence' after that lethal battle."*

—Suzann Gage, nurse practitioner, acupuncturist, nutritionist, speaker, founder/director of Progressive Health Services clinic

*"A very personal story—an easy-to-read introduction to both Western and natural medicine. **I recommend My Mother's House to non-medical people but also to doctors,** who should know how patients feel when they go through Western medicine and why they look into natural medicine."*

—Huy Hoang, MD
Natural Medical Health Center

My Mother's House

a memoir

Alexa Wolf

First Edition

First Edition

ISBN 978-0-7414-3520-0

Lanny Ostroff, cover artist.

Published by:

INFINITY PUBLISHING

1094 New DeHaven Street, Suite 100
West Conshohocken, PA 19428-2713
Info@buybooksontheweb.com
www.buybooksontheweb.com
Toll-free (877) BUY BOOK
Local Phone (610) 941-9999
Fax (610) 941-9959

Printed in the United States of America

Published January 2012

Acknowledgments

I am indebted to Barbara Heesy and Debra Killeen for reading my manuscript countless times and returning it with encouragement, editorial feedback and proofing. Eve La Salle Caram gave me endless encouragement and invaluable advice. Marcia Kerwit offered excellent editorial and proofing assistance. Constance Franklin provided unique insight. Alexis Wolfe, Cindy Haynie, Rita Martinson, and Tony Cifarelli further assisted. Jane Hoffman gave me vital publishing advice. I thank them all for their friendships as well.

I also want to thank Suzann Gage of Progressive Health Services, nurse practitioner, nutritional counselor, acupuncturist extraordinaire and dear friend for saving my life many times over. I also feel a huge appreciation for Dr. Huy Hoang for his medical assistance in recent years, Dr. Hua-Bing Wen, Cye Hoffman, Cher Lucero, Eetla Soracco, and Roger and Diana Doucette for sundry health-related assistance.

I am deeply grateful to Rita Martinson, Michael Martinson, Linda "Sam" Glynn, Sharon Longo, Laney Roberts, Janet Diamond, Maya Markota, Camilla Crachiollo, Robin Thorne, Larz Wolff, Wade Crookham, Andrew Goldsmith, Dororthy Jones (in memoriam), Karla Jones, Christine Murphy and Geralyn Motto for their friendships; plus Susan Johnson, John Rucker and again, especially, Michael Martinson, for special help.

I am indebted to my Aunt Lucy (in memoriam) and my Aunt Grace and her beloved, now deceased husband, Uncle Sid, for their love and support during the terrible months.

Finally, I want to thank Jason Wood for his extraordinary letter of encouragement early on.

Disclaimer

I have generally followed the timeframe except where the need for dramatic license, or faulty memory, intervened in my effort. I have changed some names either for legal or personal reasons.

Any nutritional or other holistic product or practice described herein is meant only to share my mother's and my story and is not intended as any kind of recommendation. Anyone interested in pursuing holistic medicine should consult with their physician.

In Memory

of

My Mother

"Into the valley of death
rode the six hundred..."

The Charge of the Light Brigade
Alfred Lord Tennyson

One of Mother's favorite poems;
the lines she often quoted.

Prologue

The House

March, 2001

Decision

I sit in the yard of my mother's house at the rusting white garden table. Rain threatens as I huddle into my coat in the cold, gray morning. Memories once more begin to revive in my flesh. Every trip here calls back my childhood and the anger of my teen years. But another reality co-exists with that time, just as visceral. It's as if there were two of Mother and two of me, our younger selves from decades ago and our loving selves from the last quarter-century, our two relationships from the two eras so different they might belong in parallel universes; and now, our last relationship, her dead self and my mourning one.

***

When I enter, my mother's house will be dark. None of the windows face the sun. Even when sunshine pours down outside and all the drapes stand open, only shadows enter. Mother never used enough wattage in the bulbs to compensate for the dimness. I don't think she wanted to spend the money, and the lack of light never bothered her. For me, however, the interior has always been too dark.

Once inside Mother's little one-story house, I will also feel some claustrophobia. Again, Mother remained blissfully unaware of any imperfection in her home. But I've always found the rooms too small and the ceiling too low, compressing and intensifying the emotional tangles between us when they existed; and, later, during our visits of love, even as the walls enveloped me in warm protection, at the same time I felt them close me in.

These days a ragged hole in the living room ceiling marks the space where a rat has returned for meals sometime since my mother's departure for her hip operation. And Mother's belongings, in mountainous welters, which I excavate and clear out on Saturdays with Susie, my friend of a decade, clog every room.

How will I manage when Susie stops helping me? I must organize Mother's business and banking files, determine what furniture I'll keep, pack those effects I want to take to my new apartment, determine what I will give friends and charities, and somehow get rid of the rest. A yard sale? But no one other than Susie has time to plow with me through the vastness of the mostly health-related periodicals piled on every flat surface, the hundreds of Mother's tapes we keep unearthing (she taped and bought tapes of political talks, relaxation meditations, health lectures and all kinds of music), so many they seem to grow out of the very walls; the countless nutritional supplements, the clothing packed into her closet so tightly that I can't move anything two inches to the side; not to mention the dishes, knick-knacks, old phones that successively stopped working, the rows of glass jars in the service porch, the numerous scissors on the kitchen table, the untold files of newspaper and health clippings that proliferated until her last moment at home—and more. The quantity of Mother's stuff is massive enough to alter gravity and warp time. (I am destined to ask Susie at least once per visit, "Have we only been at it *half-an-hour?*") After three or four Saturdays we've hardly made a dent. Driving over this morning, Susie said she won't be able to come here with me much longer.

Beneath the overcast sky, I sit in my mother's yard and fight the impulse to bolt.

Yet all this work has an ultimate goal, a question that must be resolved. Assuming I can ever get the house ready for its next occupant, who will that be? Will I live here? Or a tenant? Should I sell? What will I do with the house where I grew up, the house she owned free and clear, the house my mother loved?

Considerations

Other people's properties surround my mother's house on all sides. But a strip of land covered by a cement walkway connects her house to the street. The walkway passes along the outer edge of the yard of the house in front of Mother's, and then on through her wide wooden gate to her house.

The garden table where I sit rests on one side of the walkway, which divides her yard. Rolling along unevenly before me, it buckles over gnarled tree roots, smoothes out the last feet and stops before the three steps leading up to the deck. I am glad to sit here and not, for the moment, walk that uneven path, climb those steps.

Across from me, on the other side of the walkway, the old jacaranda dominates the yard, spangled with purple, the first blossoms of spring. More blooms lie on the ground, their petalled wimples flicking in the chilly morning breeze. I stare at them; they make me want to cry. I shift my eyes to the jacaranda. The scrubby gray-brown bark of this tree is as familiar to me as the dry skin on the back of my hand.

Beside the tree stands the decrepit tool shed built by Mitch, Mother's second husband and great love. "That tool shed isn't really legal," Mother told me. "Mitch never got a building permit." I regard the way it slumps a little, with its one small window and dark, cobwebbed interior amassed with the lamps, fixtures and other odds and ends Mitch collected from swap meets and yard sales.

I remember how, from the time Mother needed a cane, she would enter the yard and immediately detour from the dangerously cracked and heaving walkway (she couldn't risk another fall). Navigating parallel to the walkway, she passed the tree and tool shed as she trod the sparse grass, which had thinned over the years, aging with her. Where the walkway leveled out, Mother stepped onto it again and continued to the screen door of the deck.

In life she also found her own path, except at the end.

Waiting for Susie, who has dropped me off while she finds a parking space, I turn my gaze to the house. As well as building the illegal tool shed, Mitch also, as one friend recently said, "kept the house from falling down around your mother's ears." Which it began to do after he died. That is now my concern.

I consider the future and run a slew of possibilities `round my mind.

***

If I keep the house, I'll have to renovate. The roof needs to be replaced; the bathroom is moldering to the core; and, besides the rats in the ceiling, termites infest the supporting beams of the house, causing part of the foundation to list, which in turn has caused two living room windows to crack. These are just the problems of which I'm aware. Would fixing them be worth taking on major debt for the first time in my life? Could I even get a loan? And if I did, could I conjure sufficient stamina for the endless bus trips here to confirm that the construction was going as it should (as if I'd know)?

I don't drive. I always thought I'd learn when I could afford a car. Neither happened. For years it didn't matter. I had no place to go that I couldn't get to on the bus. In the last years, that circumstance changed. But there was no way I could have predicted the suffering that my inability to drive would cause my mother; and by that time it was too late. Even if I'd somehow gained access to a car, learning to drive in Los Angeles had also changed.

Cars tool through red lights, leap out of driveways into intersections and shoot across lanes without signaling, the drivers lost in their cell phone universes. Moreover, my health conditions (Rheumatoid arthritis, Chronic Fatigue Syndrome, a severe sleep disorder and an immune system that occasionally crashes due to a mysterious virus) would make my own driving dicey. My constant fatigue would inhibit the necessary attention to detail, like stop signs and other cars. I just couldn't learn to drive well enough, fast enough, to survive.

And now that same lack of skill limits my choices about the house, including the possibility of living here. Currently, most of my round trips on the bus lie west of my West Hollywood apartment. They usually require two to three hours travel. But here in Echo Park, my mother's house lies two buses and an hour-and-a-half *east* of my current starting point. To get to my doctors, dentists, friends, the clients for whom I make jewelry, and the vendors from whom I buy beads and other materials at jewelry and bead trade shows—to get there and back here to her house—would take me all day.

And what a day. The illnesses that would impair my driving proficiency exaggerate every enervating moment I undergo in the windowless, airless, occasionally cologne-drenched, often pesticide-sprayed, engine-roaring bus that is nearly always overcrowded with people and the germs they hack and sneeze into the air, air into which one climbs after an average half-hour wait, soaking in traffic noise and exhaust.

On the other hand, as one friend said, "If you sell the house, once the money is gone, it's gone. You'll never be able to afford a house after this." And she's right. And, ironically, much as I hated this house when I was younger, today I'd give anything to keep it, whether as refuge or a financial fallback position. In fact, despite the obstacles (which, besides my transportation dilemma, include forty to fifty gang members who congregate weekends at the top of the horseshoe street and have been known, if only on rare occasion, to take potshots at visitors), I dream of living here.

I could pull the carpet and restore the original hardwood floor. I could paint all the rooms, brightening them. I could install a skylight. I envision sunlight cascading into the dark living room, opening up the space. If I'm going into debt, I might as well go all the way. I could even affix solar cells to the roof and live my green dreams. And books! In my tiny bachelor apartment, the one from which I've just moved, books were stacked three-deep and lost on the dusty shelves for three decades. My new apartment, by chance one street over from the old, is a one-bedroom and big enough to build shelves. But in my mother's house, I could turn the entire smaller bedroom into my library. I could make this house truly mine, and Mother's spirit, which seems at times to move among the rooms, could remain with me.

If I lived here, I could come out onto the redwood deck, enjoying it as Mother did.

"I never noticed the birds before my cancer," Mother said, referring to her "terminal" cancer of twenty-five years before. "Now I love to sit out here and listen to them."

"The birds helped heal you."

"I'm sure they did."

Perhaps they could heal me, too.

The Deck

I turn my gaze to the deck extending out from the house. A screen encircles it. Around the screen, profusions of foliage rise up in the wild green, occasionally flowered abundance Mother loved. A multitude of birds, silent today in the damp gray morning, become on sunny days a chorus of riotous sweetness, singing from their perches in the crimson-spotted bushes, the jacaranda tree and the irregular greenery climbing the yard fence.

Through the deck screen I spy the two couches (one with a bad leg) and three lumpy rocking chairs. All are still covered, as Mother herself used to be, by the brightly colored knitted afghans friends gave her, and which she therefore treasured.

I can see her still, vivid as an exotic bird, as she sat (on the good couch) eating from the tray she brought with her and sipping with delicacy a life-saving herbal brew in her pretty china teacup.

Once of an Amazonian build, Mother's body had shrunk several octogenarian inches, but her spirit remained undiminished. Though her bones had grown fragile, her joy and fascination with life had taken on a fresh zest since her cancer, and remained robust. Her primary occupation on the deck was to read the newspaper from cover to cover, as well as various health periodicals and books, one hour vanishing into the next.

But she might also talk on the phone to me, one of her friends or her sister-in-law, Grace, with whom her friendship had continually deepened over the decades since Mother's brother, Sid, married her. Both Sid and Mother's sister, Lucy, hated the phone. You'd be lucky to get three words out of them on it. But Mother, Grace and I could talk forever. Sometimes Mother and I did, as she sat on the deck where the birds cranked out their pure joy in lilting, perfect notes; and the stereo speakers, jerry-rigged above her (a fire hazard, I've recently discovered), poured out the classical music that my mother loved (and that, inside the house, accompanied her from radio to radio as she moved from room to room).

I study the jam of wayward furniture on the deck where my mother spent so much time—the couches and rocking chairs, the ceiling-high corner cupboard, a coffee table piled with decayed periodicals, a large redwood picnic table and bench that match the redwood deck, a few rusted magazine racks overflowing with crumbling magazines, a corroded file cabinet—the lot indicative of the Herculean task within. *What a packrat!* I tell her, and smile.

I feel Mother laughing with me. For a moment, behind her imagined companionable laughter, I hear an echo of the great guffaw for which she was famous among her friends, one reason they loved her so. *AHHH—hahahahahahahaaaa!*

"I can't die now," she used to say, procrastinating the hip replacement surgery she needed, with its risk. "I'd be embarrassed to leave you with all this."

My smile falls away.

A stillness lies over the deck this morning, an enchantment of eternal sleep, although whether a peaceful or terrible enchantment I cannot say.

Spells

Mother determined that if she survived her hip operation and was able to walk again without pain and the other physical limitations her bad hip imposed, she could return home and live alone, independently, the way she wanted. But she added that if she died on the table, so be it. "Don't feel bad," she tried to comfort me in advance. "I've had a good life."

She survived the surgery. All that remained for her was to learn to walk again at the skilled nursing care hospital. After that, she'd go home, where she would require further assistance for another few months. Then, at last, she would again possess her autonomy and privacy, her deck and her newspaper and the sound of the birds and the music.

Today people comment, "Well, tsk, tsk, tsk about the way she died, but after all she was eighty-six," as if the particular joys of an older person are a lesser experience than those of someone younger, indeed, as if their life itself is worth less. But the elderly themselves do not express this view. I do know many who prefer death to the kind of "care" they'll find as their bodies break down, the "care" my mother underwent. I too would rather be dead. But my mother loved life. Even a few days on her terms—with a little money and living at home on her own—let alone a few or several more years, however imperfect, would have been a great gift.

But it was a gift she was not to receive.

At the time, people warned me about the hospital. "You have to be there." I didn't believe it. Be there or what? If you don't personally watch the people who are supposed to be saving your loved one, they'll kill her?

But the warnings were valid. This common operation catapulted my mother into the nursing care system. "Rack and ruin!" she herself might have called it; indeed, I can hear her in my mind. "RACK AND ***RU-IN!***" my literary, dramatic, ironic mother would have enunciated her fate with a flamboyance possible only before her "caretakers" got their hands on her.

For I couldn't visit her often enough, and I missed the mounting realities. I kept falling beneath the spokes of the colossal wheel of inhumanity that kept rolling over Mother and me and grinding us both under. That is how her singular path ended.

And I cannot get past it.

I need to remember and honor the hell my mother endured and yet not get mired in that memory. But where do you find in the death of a loved one, especially an awful and unnecessary death, a way to accept and transcend it? A lethargy of spirit pervades my will. I can't seem to move forward on anything. I should at least call an exterminator for the rats and termites. But with everything the house needs, why start there? Or stop there, for that matter. I feel as if I've wandered into a fairytale, a story of sorcery in which the heroine looks into the eyes of the wicked witch and they turn her to stone.

I sometimes think, of everything, *What's the point?*

Stone.

***

Everything remains to be done, including making the decision, an achievement which seems more distant than ever. And while I dawdle, I am anxious lest a vagrant slip into the unoccupied building and set it on fire, an earthquake shake it to the ground or the housing bubble burst before I can sell it, if that's what I finally choose to do. But how can I decide?

How can I let the house go? At the same time it announces my mother is not coming back, it embraces and harbors her spirit.

Yet as much as I resist selling it, I resist even more entering. I need my memories. But I don't want to face them. Perhaps I somehow think that if I keep the house, I can avoid the pain of remembering. The house will keep my memories, good and bad.

Sharon, my friend since junior high, who was present from the beginning of Mother's and my metamorphoses, said recently, "At least you were able to have a loving relationship with her before she died." But for that very reason, a little voice within me cries out in dazed bewilderment, *Where is my mommy? When is Mommy coming home?* And I have to give my child self the same answer I silently gave my mother when she lay awash in drugs and dementias, unable ever to walk again. "When can I go home?" she asked me at each visit. *Never. You're never going home.*

I'm still rocking in the aftermath of her death four months ago.

I stand and look down the walkway. No sign of Susie. I feel profound relief at this opportunity to delay going inside. For my mother's house, when I come here, still closes me in, with its darkness, its too-low ceiling and too-small rooms, and its wraiths of recollection from all our shared eras, Mother's and mine, bumping into each other in the ambience both loving and suffocating that wraps itself around me the moment I enter.

Book One

Family

1963 to 1965

A Demand

"What did I ever do that was so terrible?" Mother demanded to know when I was nineteen. A couple of months before, I'd nearly plunged a knife into her. Now she was driving me and another load of my belongings to my first apartment, helping me move out of her house for good.

A cornucopia of possible answers spilled forth into my mind and spread themselves luxuriantly before me. My mother possessed myriad dictatorial stratagems ranging from the dismissive wave of her hand and tone of voice, to her obsessive scrutiny of everything that was wrong with me, to her demand for every last piece of my soul.

"Why are you so angry?" she persevered.

Her very question made me so angry I could spit acid.

One day I would be that angry on her behalf. But that day lay decades in the future. Indeed, it astounds me that we ever reached it; that we even managed our death-defying ride past the nightmarish knife-wielding moment from which Mother's demand for explanation arose, let alone that we eventually developed so close and loving a friendship. For, looking back at what I still consider my mother's narcissistic, slightly insane behavior during my childhood and teens, and my particular personality traits that caused me to react to her as I did, I cannot help but shudder: Not only ourselves but our family history dictated our nearly fatal collision.

The Best of Them

Mother was the oldest of three children: Sid, Lucy and my mother herself. Lucy became a slender gorgeous blonde who in her early twenties, in the picture I have of her, looks like Lauren Bacall. My mother, by contrast, had weight problems since her teens. Ranging between sizes fourteen and sixteen, depending on the clothing brand and her diet at the moment, she averaged twenty-five pounds over her optimum weight until her seventies, when she became chronically underweight. She also had acne as a teen. ("In those days," she told me, "they treated acne with radiation." Fields of skin cancers migrated across her face in her senior years.) Mother grew up seeing herself as the unattractive one, a self-image shc carried most of her life. But she persisted in making herself as attractive and interesting as possible.

She hennaed her hair, becoming a redhead in order to stand out from others, especially (or so I guess) her beautiful blonde sister. She read all manner of books on health and beauty and utilized what she learned, just as decades later she would utilize all she discovered about holistic medicine to save herself from "terminal" cancer. For beauty's sake, she rubbed her hands with lemon peel after doing dishes, spread mayonnaise on her face at night and concocted a vinegar and water solution to pour over herself after showers to restore "the acid mantle." She went on countless diets and once purchased a machine with a wide strap that went across her buttocks and gyrated.

This machine was supposed to whip off all that blubber. I witnessed its initiation. Mother stepped onto the device (the base of it appropriately looking like a weight scale), buckled the strap in place across her behind, flipped the "on" switch and, with typical gusto, threw herself back against the strap before the engine was fully on. The strap whipped once. Then, with a whine and a groan, the engine stopped dead, never to be revived.

Yet except for her weight, the photograph I once had of my mother (and placed in a safe place and thereby lost forever), from *her* early twenties, revealed her appearance to be that of a young Katharine Hepburn. Her similar facial contours included the high cheekbones, delicate straight nose and well-shaped expressive eyes (Mother's were brown). Mother was every bit as beautiful as Lucy. Her insecurity about her looks came mostly from her mother. My maternal grandmother always introduced the three children like this: "This is Horty, Sid and Lucy, and Lucy is thebestofthem," the last and defining words running together as a single adjective.

I was in my teens the first time Mother described these unvarying introductions. I'd recently begun therapy. A conversation between Mother and myself about my sessions must have triggered Mother's memory. "How did you feel about that?" I asked. Although the trouble between us was nearing its zenith, I was stunned for Mother's sake.

"I didn't think anything of it."

I was dumbfounded. *"'And Lucy is 'the best of them'?* Didn't you feel *horrible?*"

"I don't remember feeling anything."

"But now?" I queried. "What do you feel now?"

"I don't know." She thought about it. "I don't think I feel anything. I just didn't think anything of it."

Decades after that conversation, when my mother and I had become friends, I asked her again, more than once, about her feelings regarding her mother demeaning her, although I didn't use the word "demeaning." But despite my urging and probing, even after she'd made so many other transformations, Mother remained unaware of any pain connected with having heard her own mother present her younger sister to everyone as "the best of them." In fact, Mother had managed to continue repressing her pain despite the fact that life itself seemed to rub in her mother's description.

My father attempted to become an actor, failed, then worked as a fencing master; and he gambled. Mother divorced him when I was one or two because of his gambling.

Lucy, on the other hand, married Roland Kibbee, a big muckety-muck writer-producer at Universal Studios who made a ton of money. Lucy's and Kibb's marriage was good and lasted decades, until he died.

Kibb was also Burt Lancaster's best friend. My grandmother kept a signed photo of a smiling Lancaster on her living room table. "He drove me home from Lucy's last week," she would brag, puzzling me as I glanced at the photograph. To my child's mind, movie star or not, this was a man with way too many teeth. Mother never met him. (I did in my early forties, under strikingly unpredictable circumstances: I introduced myself to him at a fund-raiser for AIDS, the virus for which I was, at the time, misdiagnosed.)

When I was a child, Mother and I went to Lucy's and Kibb's house every Thanksgiving. An only child, I loved playing with my three cousins and being around my aunt and uncle. This was a real family of which I became a part, as opposed to just Mother and me. But for some reason Mother never explained, those enjoyable family get-togethers stopped when I was seven or eight, and Lucy and Mother lost intimacy for decades.

However, when Mother got cancer, Lucy visited her and the two sisters began speaking periodically on the phone. "Lucy is going to send me a hundred dollars a month to pay Isela," Mother told me with affection and pride. Isela was Mother's housekeeper and yard keeper as well as friend and neighbor. The sisters' love had not been that strong since they were young.

When Mother was in the hospital after her hip surgery, Lucy and I spoke briefly on the phone a couple times a month. Like Grace, Mother's sister-in-law, with whom I spoke every night, Lucy could not have been more supportive. "You're a rock," she told me when Mother's pain and helplessness had totally demoralized her and I felt my most useless.

Considering Lucy's wealth, I suspect Mother's disdain for materialism hurt their earlier relationship. Her attitude came from her leftist politics, or so I once thought. But my mother's disparagement of material values was matched only by her fear of poverty. Her father had died when she was twelve, and she watched her own mother—"one of the first Jewish nurses in the country," she announced—struggle to support three children. It must have been a savage battle, imprinting itself upon Mother's deepest psyche and, in a sometimes humiliating fashion, mine.

Once in my early teens, after I blew my nose and tossed the Kleenex, Mother bestowed upon me one of her furiously anxious frowns, raced around me into the bathroom, snatched up my used Kleenex from the wastepaper basket, opened it to inspect what I'd produced, and exclaimed, "You didn't use all of this Kleenex! You wasted some of it! Use it *all* before you throw it away!"

During our recent years of loving communication, I asked her, "Do you ever dream?" I'd been fascinated by my own dreams since my teens.

"Well." She searched her mind. "Sometimes I dream someone stole my purse." Even in her dreams she feared poverty. But that was not the worst example.

Last year, when she lay in the hospital submerged and drifting in morphine and other drugs, she said, "Oh, call me! I don't care if I'm asleep. I always want to talk to you. Don't worry about waking me up." But the next time I phoned, she swam out of sleep in a panicked delusion. "I don't owe any rent! I paid my rent! I don't owe any money!" That was the last call I made without checking with the nurse's station first to make sure my mother was awake.

But Mother was a good person. That was one of her great character assets and also her self-image. How could she admit envy for her successful sister?

However, there was another story concerning Mother and Lucy. About *that* story Mother did possess emotional clarity. My grandmother had apparently determined that when Lucy wasn't "the best of them," Lucy would be made the best.

The Essay

After Mother graduated from high school and found a job, her high school announced an essay contest. Lucy, two years younger than Mother, still attended the school. While Aunt Lucy was very smart, Mother was the one who possessed the writing gift.

"Mother told me to write an essay for Lucy," my mother related to me, "and she told Lucy to enter the essay in the contest under her own name."

"But that's terrible." Her mother was ruthlessly using her to build up Lucy.

"Lucy didn't want to do it, either. She didn't want to use my essay. Neither of us wanted to do it. But my mother insisted."

My mother's mother possessed tremendous inner strength. But a streak of tyranny runs through our family. Ahma, as I called my grandmother, had escaped an abusive father who drove her sister, a grandaunt I never met, into a mental hospital. There, as far as I know, Ahma's sister died. Ahma left home as soon as she could and made a good marriage. Mother told me, "My father was the most wonderful man. He was so kind to everyone. We all adored him."

But he died when Mother was twelve, and after his death (or perhaps before; I never knew), my grandmother's strength crossed over into something darker. She carried within herself her father's dictatorial character. "Mind me. I know best." It was her most frequent edict. When Mother's high school announced the essay contest, my grandmother said it again. Both girls minded her. Mother wrote the essay. Lucy submitted it in her own name.

Mother's essay won the contest. Now the sisters were stuck with the results. Mother went to the lunch that celebrated Lucy "winning." Both girls were miserable.

A few years ago Mother added something to the story. "My mother didn't remember that I wrote the essay. She forgot she made me." Her mother had died thirty-some years before. "She forgot she ordered me to do it. Now Lucy's forgotten, too." This time when Mother spoke, I heard pain limned by anger.

At the lunch that celebrated Lucy "winning" the contest, the school principal said to Mother, "You're one of the brightest students we've ever had." Yet she never suggested my mother attend college and develop a career, and it never occurred to my mother, despite her intense desire to be a writer.

My father told me that when he met her, "Your mother used to literally run home from the bus so she could write." However, she went to work right out of high school, earning money in a C.B. DeMille extravaganza, the name of which I never thought to ask. But she once showed me a picture of herself standing on a ledge in shorts and a halter-top posing as an Amazon with a line of other extras. That movie was where she met my father.

If not a writer, Mother might have become an excellent photographer. She kept a camera with her for years, snapping whatever snagged her distinctive imagination. Once, on her way to her car after leaving her office in downtown Los Angeles, she passed a lot where a building had been torn down. "Everything was in rubble," she told me that night, and breathed in remembered awe, "It was like the end of the world. And there right in the middle of it stood this piano." She showed me the pictures she'd taken of it. It did look like the end of the world.

The law also fascinated her. But instead of becoming the brilliant lawyer that lay within her capability, Mother followed her job as a movie extra with a job as a transcriber. She settled into typing from a Dictaphone the transcripts of civil trials provided her by court reporters.

What became of her aspirations to write? With the exception of one poem she unearthed in her last few years and gave me, her transcriber job supplied material for her only other surviving literary effort. Mother excerpted verbatim the humorous exchanges she found in the transcripts she typed, and compiled them into a book. She gave me a copy years ago, which I promptly mislaid. I always planned to get another from her. Today I will again search within her house, a bit feverishly, for the folder that holds her copies of her one book.

Despite her high school principal's praise, it was not an era for women. After her graduation, Mother had just kept working, blind to any career prospects. She also continued to denigrate materialism while, simultaneously, for the rest of her life, she carried a dread of falling into poverty.

Even during my late teens, when I hated my mother, I knew these stories and a part of me sympathized with her. Mother's earlier life explained a lot of her behavior. Looking back today I understand her still better. When I was a teen, my adolescent hormones were on a trapeze. But Mother bore me when she was thirty-one. When I was a teen my mother may have been in peri-menopause, bouncing around in her own hormonal imbalances.

Moreover, from the time she divorced my father, she was wont to exclaim, "I have to be both mother and father to you."

No you don't! I would think, dryly and with force, wishing my father were there to afford a refuge from the obsessive intensity my mother fixated upon me. But within a year after their divorce my father went to Mexico, where he lived for ten years.

Of course, if my father had paid Mother any alimony, it would have eased her stress. Instead, she had to support us both. She told me in our good years, "I was terrified I would fail." So Mother had all these stresses pressing upon her, bringing up a child alone with no emotional or financial support, and she'd never felt good about herself. She was in a pressure cooker.

But so, at the same time, was I.

And yet—what *did* she do to inspire the wrath I'd exhibited? No one looking at us could have understood my anger, had they known of it, any more than she did. Did she not, when I was little, place a second door handle lower on the door so I could reach it easily and not feel intimidated? Didn't she watch all my television shows with me? Didn't she take me to see Mary Martin in the *Peter Pan* musical *twice* because I loved it so much? Didn't she, among other things, attempt to convince me, in my feeling of being so ugly, that I was the classical Ugly Duckling who was really a swan? And when that logic failed, didn't she make sacrifices to rescue me from my unhappiness?

Dress Rehearsals

"Big Nose!" "Long Nose!" taunted the other grammar school children, rejecting me from their game. I must have been angry, yet all I consciously felt was shame and hurt and that they were right.

Yes, that *nose*, with its big hump below the bridge, its length, its hook, the excessive size: it was my father's nose. I could see from photographs that it was attractive on him. But it stood out on my thin face, abnormal and ugly, just as I stood outside the circle of children linking hands and mocking me.

I smiled back at them as if to say, *Yes, I agree with you, see, I don't like me either. You don't have to attack me.* I hated myself for that self-demeaning smile. But I continued to splash it across my face at their daily derisions. I didn't know what else to do. I came home crying every day, burning with the shame of not being worthy of them and their knowing it.

When Mother got home from work at night and heard my sad stories, she buried me in a gigantic hug of love and concern. Bosom overflowing with sympathy, she comforted, "It's all right, dear. It's all right. They're all terrible."

Mother had begun shielding me from life much earlier. One day during a dinner with Alta, Mother's closest friend, Alta told me, "When you were a toddler, your mother kept pillows in the car trunk. She was always spreading them around you."

Mother said to Alta, "But if she fell, I didn't want her to hurt herself!"

Alta laughed. "Your mother is a real character," she told me recently. She never got over those pillows.

Sometimes I've imagined a different mother, perhaps also a character, but perhaps also impossibly wise, advising me, when the other children called me names, "But you have friends who do like you." Notably Laney, Alta's daughter; we were born five days apart. Alta and my mother met in the hospital while giving birth to us; and just as Mother and Alta remained friends for life, so would Laney and I. Manuel, who lived in the house in front, was another good friend. We pulled each other around in my little red wagon when we were little. Later, when we were older, we ran all over the hill that, starting at the top of our horseshoe street, rose up above our houses. After Mother took me to see *Peter Pan*, I collected Manuel and two other neighborhood kids to re-enact the play with me. Manuel and I also replayed scenes from science fiction movies we saw together at the local theater. I screamed as imaginary monsters assailed us, and he saved me.

"Some people," a perfect Mother might have told me, "will like you and some won't. Some people will be your friends and some won't. Just be a good friend to those who are."

Instead, however, in my teens, she commenced a different refrain of comforting words. Whenever some adolescent disaster befell me (like a bad date or, much more often, no date), she said, "That isn't life, dear. It's just a dress rehearsal." She cast "dress rehearsals" around me like those pillows in my toddlerhood, to relieve whatever pain I was undergoing.

But the pain from which she tried to spare me was usually a pain that couldn't be avoided, it could only be felt, understood and gotten through. Rather than helping me learn from it, Mother's "dress rehearsals," though born of love, invalidated my experience, eviscerated my sense of reality, undermined my potential strength and, to my mind, broadcast the message that she had to protect me from reality because I was incapable of dealing with it myself.

Meanwhile, if the Scylla of her overprotection beset me on one side, on the other loomed the Charybdis of verbal abuse. That's where I learned my self-hating smile.

The Smile

"Smile or people won't like you!" Mother admonished. If I didn't smile, Other People wouldn't like me, and it would be my fault. Worse, it would reflect upon Mother, although she never voiced or even recognized this underlying motive.

So I smiled to please her. I smiled because it was the only way I knew to make Other People like me. I smiled my Good Little Girl smile, my placating smile, I smiled the smile that said, *Yes, I don't think much of me, either, so that puts us on the same side. Right?* And then, entering my teens, and clear through my twenties, I found myself smiling without volition. A compulsive smile confiscated control of my face whenever rejection, real or imaginary, threatened.

I perceived rejection when I was about to stand up for myself in some minor way, and I expected the other person to reject me for such an act of insurgency—what right did I have to stand up for myself to good-enough Other People? Or I might anticipate rejection simply because I was me and dared, nonetheless, to exist. I smiled and despised my smile and loathed myself for producing it.

I was unaware that most mothers admonished their daughters to smile; rather like slave parents must have inculcated in their children the need to smile around the white male power structure. *Make sure they know you are happy, and submissive in your role,* ***and not a threat.*** This historical reality made my mother's injunction to smile also an act of love, however perverse.

But my occasional failure to smile, my momentary forgetfulness or, later, rebellion, comprised only one of the many subsets of my core wrongness.

"There's something *radically wronggg* with you!" Mother accused me. "What's *wronggg* with you?" she interrogated like a lawyer in one of her transcripts. "Tell me!" Then she would wait, expectant and impatient, her brows bunched with anxiety, her eyes boring into me for answers. I didn't know how to respond. What *was* wrong with me? She loved me. She was always telling me she loved me. How could I do this to her (whatever *this* was at any given moment)?

My radical wrongness nauseated me. But except for sometimes failing to smile, I never knew what might inspire her charge, only that she delivered it in wild unpredictable bursts, and in many variations, with the same shocked horror and terror every time. A "radical wrongness" contaminated me. This was the central fact that she drilled into me with histrionic verbiage and supercharged emotions, and that in my late teens would cause me to erupt in blinding rage.

A Few Subsets

But my anger began much earlier.

"I hate you, I hate you!" I screamed when I was six.

"Oh, you don't hate me. You really love me," Mother said in a knowing voice. "Here, dear." She tossed me a pillow. "Hit this pillow and pretend it's me."

I screamed again. But in reality only an impotent whimper of my fury remained, a ghost in the sudden emotional void inside me. I didn't hate her. I loved her. She knew. I didn't. Only Mother knew what I *really* felt—and wanted, thought, perceived; a knowledge that increased through the years.

"Oh, you don't want this," she would say, of something for which I'd just asked. "You don't believe this," of whatever I'd just said. "Oh, you just imagined that," of something I remembered. "You don't mean that," about whatever I meant. "You don't need a new blouse," of the one grown too small, until *she* saw it on me and confirmed for herself it didn't fit.

I didn't know it, mean it, want it, believe it, feel it, think it, or need it unless she believed and acknowledged that I did; and if I insisted on expressing my true feelings, if I did think it, feel it, want it—if I continued to trust my experience of reality, there was something *radically wrong* with me.

Paradoxically, the more Mother undermined my self-confidence, the more I needed her to validate precisely what I no longer trusted in myself, and I despised my neediness.

Simultaneously, in another part of myself, I condemned her for these fervent exclamations of disappointment in me. In my heart a hard accretion of fury toward her was forming.

"You failed me, you failed me!" Mother howled, producing another of her frequent, horrified reiterations when I unknowingly exposed my to-the-roots wrongness.

(Had I giggled with my hand over my mouth? "Take your hand away from your mouth!" Had I not smiled at someone? Had I forgotten to brush my teeth?) I cowered away from her, sickened by shame. Then I discovered what I expected would prove a defense against this particular attack.

By age eight I'd read the popular book, *The Fifty-Minute Hour*, written by a psychologist. I'd also read *The Snake Pit* and seen the movie on TV. These two resources gave me a precocious awareness of psychology. One day when Mother let me know I'd failed her, I volleyed back, "That's not something you should tell a child."

Caught off guard, she thought a moment, processed this insight and came to agreement. My mother then wailed, right on cue, "I failed you! I failed you!"

Not only could I find no way around her attacks, she always seemed to take my wrongness to a new level. Shortly after my menstruation began, on a Jewish holiday, I sat in the back seat of the car with Ahma, my grandmother, as Mother drove us to meet Alta's and Grace's family at Temple. We were going to be amongst Other People. Not good.

My period, only my third or fourth, had begun that morning. Wearing a starched, light-colored dress, I was unnerved by the heavy flow of blood. My lower abdomen throbbed with pain. A dull dread fluttered in my heart. I looked out the open car window as we drove. Cool air blew over my hot face. What if blood leaked through my dress? The blood was disgusting and there was so much of it. I felt like a heavy, sodden blob of mindless fatigue and cramping pain that might loose a degrading red river into my clothes from my vagina. People would know I was disgusting to my fundamental female being.

Glancing back at me in her rearview mirror, Mother underwent a change. In the instant it took her to focus on me, her brows flew up in shock and anger. Her mouth popped open in a gasp. The high-pitched anxiety that always seemed to prowl the margins of her personality as well as her voice exploded full-blown into the horror and terror I always seemed to ignite in her. Swiveling sharply forward again, her eyes on traffic, she brandished one of her best, characteristically descriptive passages with an irrepressible linguistic flamboyance that hammered me flat.

"Oh my God! *Smile!* What's ***wrong*** with you? You look like a gloomy, damp, dank, dark, UGLY ***THUNDERCLOUD!"***

Every word sent me shriveling farther into myself. By the time she hit the grand finale noun, I had sealed myself up for the day into a closed ball of gloomy, dank, dark, ugly, humiliated anger, about a hundred times more depressed than I'd been the moment before.

But it was the incident with the snake that commenced a nightmare whose imagery summed up my entire inner life and predicted, to a degree, my outer life to come. The whole thing was about love. That's why it impacted me so powerfully.

The Snake

I was an infant when my mother and father gave me a Siamese kitten and nine when my allergy doctor told Mother I had to give him up. I lost my best friend of all, my feline sibling, and the doctor forbade me any other animal with hair, fur or feathers. But one day when I was twelve a neighborhood boy caught a garden snake. I stroked its back with my forefinger while it wound itself around the boy's hand. Sensing an intelligent if alien life pulsing through the reptile, I was certain that if I had a snake, it would know me and, in its own snaky way, love me.

That night, bursting with excitement, I asked Mother if I could have a snake. It never dawned on me she might refuse. But, cooking a Polynesian chicken dish, she nearly tossed the rice and raisins from the ladle when she threw up her hands. "Oh my God, people will think you are WEIRD!"

Familiar nausea whipped through my gut. I was a failure, wrong to my very roots and now, longing for a pet, *weird.* But Mother must have decided I could have a snake after all because, in the next scene I recall, we are sitting in the living room looking in the yellow pages. I'm literally bouncing on the couch with joy. I'm going to get a snake! *I'm going to have a pet to love.* I point to a large, bordered advertisement for a pet store. "Look! They sell snakes!"

Mother looks. She looks harder. She exclaims, "Oh my god. Your *fingernails!"* My eyes flick uncontrollably to my fingernails. Mother says, "They're long and yellow and curling—just like *those old women down at* ***Angel's Flight!!!"***

I jerk my glance back from my disgusting, bag-lady fingernails, which I whisk back to my lap.

Yet Mother did take me to a pet store. I remember trotting ahead of her along the walkway en route to her car when she suddenly observed, "You're walking with your feet out! You're walking like a ***duck!*** You're walking **JUST LIKE YOUR *FATHER!*"**

For an instant, gone before I could fully record it in my consciousness, my heart seemed to implode with its own worthlessness. It was all hopeless, my attempt to please her, to take joy in bits of life, just to live. I couldn't *walk* without revealing my innate wrongness.

How beautiful was that black snake in the store with its undulations, rising off the broad, hairy wrist of the store owner who showed it to me. But I didn't take the graceful creature home. I couldn't even bring myself to touch it. The very thought terrified me. My excitement at finding an animal that, despite my allergies, could be a pet and soothe my loneliness, had transmogrified into fear—and nightmare.

A seething mass of snakes covers our yard. They hang from the jacaranda tree and swarm over the deck. They are writhing, fanged and poisonous; and in dream after dream I stand petrified before them, at the gate to our yard, unable to take another step. The nightmare snakes will not let me go home. They'll kill me. I can't get back to "where I live."

I can't get back to myself. The path is poisoned.

For years I wouldn't know how to get "home;" and then, years after I found my way, another abusive living situation would wear me down and I'd lose myself again just when Mother, having become my loving friend, was in her own hell and most needed me to be strong for her.

***

I read more psychology, discovered the term "psychosomatic," decided that was the nature of my allergies, and they went away. The next year, when I was fourteen, I got a dog. And started high school. Things were going to be different there. Somehow. I was going to be happy. Life was opening up. I felt a tremendous excitement although the snake nightmares persisted; and I still had that nose.

Dumbo

Long Nose, Big Nose. My father's nose. If only I'd inherited his wavy black hair instead. According to his mother, in the one conversation I ever had with her—she lived somewhere "back East" in a nursing home, a fact which held no meaning for me then—she told me our family had lived in Spain in the 16th Century. If only Father's black, wavy, Spanish hair framed my too-thin countenance and enhanced my too-narrow hazel eyes, as opposed to the nondescript brunette that was my fare, along with my duck feet, bag-lady fingernails and underused Kleenex!

But somewhere between Mother's overprotection and hysterical verbal abuse ran the true spirit of her love. She encouraged mc to feel good about myself. "Your nose is your Dumbo," she said. I immediately understood her symbolism although today it baffles me. Dumbo had big ears and the other animals made fun of him. Then he learned to fly with his ears. So...Dumbo's big ears were his humiliating flaw but they turned out to be the source of his flying gift? I'd fly even with my nose if I just accepted it? My Inner Beauty lay in the hump and hook of my nose, the very object of people's disdain?

Well, whatever the symbolism, although I might intellectually have agreed with it, I knew I was ugly and waited with desperate impatience until at sixteen I was old enough for a "nose job." Mother scraped the money together. Ahma, the nurse, found a doctor. I was going to be pretty.

But Sharon, my best friend, was beautiful. Fashioning a stylish "beehive," she piled her long blonde hair high inches atop her head, sprayed it until it petrified and curled the remainder below her neck. Men buzzed around her. My new ski jump-tilted nose couldn't compete.

To set myself apart, I scissored my hair into a pixie cut and hennaed it. But the coppery red only emphasized the innate jaundice-yellow shade in my skin and enticed no parade of heroes to throw themselves at my feet. Forget red. Blondes had more fun. I got a bottle of blonde dye from a drugstore. Unfortunately, it turned my henna-red hair neon orange, thereby setting me several unexpected decades ahead of my time (and definitely apart from Sharon). Growing it out took a full semester.

Mother, unpredictably, found nothing amiss with my hair color. Instead, having given me a new nose, she now enabled me to pursue another part of the life I wanted to live.

Actress

With a new nose on my face and my orange hair back to henna-red, my confidence scaled upward, permitting something pivotal to occur.

In grammar school I'd loved drawing pictures, especially using crayons for our map assignments. Mother sent all my pictures, maps and report cards to my father in Mexico, or so she told me. He did not respond. But I felt good that he knew what was happening in my life. It was almost as if he were with me.

I also liked to write. When I was ten, I entered a poetry contest for my age group sponsored by the Women's International League for Peace and Freedom. When an envelope arrived from them a few months later, I had such a good feeling about it that I was afraid to dare hope. Yet hope I did. Yet what happened overwhelmed me nonetheless. Opening the envelope, I extracted the typed page within. Upon it I saw my name next to the words, "First Place."

My head swam with incredulous joy. Euphoria swept through me. *I won.* A check for fifteen dollars accompanied a book by Albert Einstein called *Peace or Atomic War?* Glory intoxicated me for days. I made a photocopy of the check, nailed it to my bedroom door and kept it for years. I still have the book.

But my greatest passion was acting. Ever since grammar school, I took acting classes. That's where I felt my true gift lay. I was not a popular girl and did not get roles in the school plays. But when I was sixteen and had a new nose, Mother took me to a local performance of *Hamlet.* Afterwards I wanted to say hello to the star, Guy Stockwell, a stunningly handsome and talented actor. I was nervous and ready to leave but Mother accompanied me to the well-lit theater patio where the actors came out to greet their audience in the summer night. I found Guy and told him how much I liked his performance. He introduced me to Don Freed, the play's director. Don would one day go on to become a multiple award-winning playwright. Don and Guy had co-founded the Los Angeles Art Theater (LAAT), the repertory company that had just put on the Shakespearean classic. "Why don't you join the theater?" Don invited me. "You'd be more than welcome."

Thrilled, I looked at Mother. She agreed to pay the small fee and drive me each week to the upstairs room in the small two-story West Hollywood building where the theater company met.

At sixteen, I was the youngest member of the group. Everyone else, at least in their twenties, was gracious and respectful, a totally singular experience for me. Singer Gale Garnett was particularly kind, welcoming me the first day with a warm smile, surprising me by knowing my name. Each week I performed voice and diction, physical exercises and improvisations with the grown-up professionals, loving every second.

I couldn't have gone there without Mother's help.

Within a few months I got the lead in a children's production of *Around the World in 80 Days*. Mother drove me to all the evening rehearsals.

Parallel Stages

Actually, the director had cast his girlfriend as the lead, the Indian princess, but they had a fight. He waited an hour for her to show up to start rehearsals. I was there as an understudy. I got the role by default. But I got the role. Don played the male lead. Rehearsals with him revealed that the intermittent, incandescent, intuitive glimpses about acting I'd had in the past were correct. Acting could help me overcome the emotional problems that had begun to swarm through me.

As an actor your emotions lie near the surface. Partially through your character's dialogue, you express those emotions.

By contrast, in real life I was often speechless. Someone would say or do something, and my mind tortured itself over whether I was right to feel what I felt about it and whether to do or say what my emotions prompted me to do or say. If I did choose to verbalize a feeling or thought, I still stalled, working out how to phrase it, reviewing how the Other Person or Other People might respond to me and how I, in turn, might protect myself from their almost assuredly negative response to me. If someone slighted me, my self-examination over the accuracy of my insulted feelings could go on for two years before I brought those feelings to the other person to discuss. Meanwhile, I smiled. This did not endear me to others.

As an actor you listen to the other actors and move on instinct, reacting without inhibition. But it had always been a spontaneous comment or act that roused Mother's horror and terror. In my real life I no longer reacted spontaneously to anything. I never trusted or acted on my instincts. I'd feel anger, curiosity, sorrow. But I would smile my compulsive smile, my Please Like Me smile, my Good Little Girl smile, my smile of self-hatred, while my true self lay like a mastodon buried for eons beneath the glacial reality of that false smile.

However, as an actress I'd dare to experiment and be spontaneous, then make clear choices and trust them. "Be audacious!" instructed one of Don's assistant teachers. I loved this! I knew that once I decided what the character I played would do, I would audaciously act out that decision. I was certain that, feeling secure as someone else, I would animate my characters' inner life from the subtlest daubs of emotion and sensation to the boldest strokes of feeling. Then I'd bring these theatrical experiences and feelings into my real life.

By discovering and letting my characters' inmost selves emerge, as I nurtured and elaborated the personalities of one character after another, I would pull up the parts of myself too wounded to surface on their own or even to see. As an actor I would love my characters' feelings, choices, eccentricities, mistakes, successes, instincts, and uniqueness. Through acting them out on stage, I would come to love my own.

Finally, as Don taught us at the LAAT, to be powerful on stage or on the screen, you maintain a reserve of feeling. No matter how much emotion an actor reveals through their character, the audience has to sense more, so intense and deep it would be impossible for the character to express it all. This fathomless well of raw but undischarged emotion creates an aura of charisma and compels the audience. I would do this. Beyond what a character knew or was able to express, I would let simmer an inexpressible depth of feeling, thus centering myself in an otherwise unobtainable personal power; knowing my roots instead of being contaminated by Mother's view of them. This was how I'd overcome the emotional torques and teen torments I found at home.

No matter how tired she was, Mother drove me to rehearsals at night, enthusiastically supporting my love of acting and, when the time came, excited by my performance. Our *Around the World* production played two weekend afternoons at the Coronet Theater, received no reviews and gave me a taste of what my life could become.

I'd often sensed an ability in myself to command the stage. Nothing special occurred in my Coronet Theater debut to confirm that potential. Yet I felt that portraying the Indian princess was preparing me to succeed at what I loved most.

Mother totally supported me in my anticipation of becoming an acting success. Yet at the same time her erratic but recurrent repudiations of my deepest self, repudiations which lay on the other side of all her support for my creativity and of all her endearments, shaped the rage building as a pressure in my head and poison in my heart because, except in the LAAT, I believed Mother's most negative edition of myself.

Performance

During the next semester at high school I hit the first true rung of my acting ability. The theater department teacher decided to present a series of scenes for the school instead of a play. I joined up with Carol, another unpopular actress. We chose twenty minutes from the play, *The Heiress.* I took the starring role, portraying the young woman betrayed by her lover.

On the night of the performance, I repeated the neurotic pattern I'd begun to develop during *Around the World.* First I let myself become a wreck. Was I good enough? Could I do this? What if I was terrible? Somehow questioning myself in this negative manner stimulated my energy. I drew that energy into my solar plexus and let it spread until it filled me. Then, ejecting self-doubt, I centered myself in the energy and the character.

When I walked on stage as the heroine of the play, I could feel my magnetism. I could feel the magic. And all the work I'd done on the character, the many rehearsals experimenting with her, made her vital. As the scene progressed, I could feel the audience sharing my feelings. I sensed their tension and held breath. During the most dramatic moment, when the other character slapped me, I heard someone in the audience gasp.

None of the other students in the theater department bothered to watch Carol and me. The teacher didn't know we existed. He had his pets and neither of us was one of them. In fact, I wonder how we even managed to get permission to perform our scene. But afterwards Mother told me with pride, "I saw three or four women with tears in their eyes."

"Really?"

"Oh, yes. You were *wonderful.*"

And I felt the truth bouncing back from her. She wasn't just a deluded, bragging mother. I'd done it. I knew irrevocably it was true. This had been my goal since my first impulse toward acting drove me to organize Manuel and the other neighborhood kids to play *Peter Pan* with me and act out science fiction monster movie scenes. I had talent. I could be an actress. I was good. *This is what I was meant to do. I can do it!*

Then my eating disorder, which had begun a few years earlier, flared up. Eventually, it was my compulsive eating that would spark Mother's and my tinderbox of madness.

Food

Chocolate-covered raisins, eaten at movies when I was a child; the unbearable sleepiness immediately after finishing; the doctor who ignored my description of this strange slumber; grabbing another box at the next movie: this was the beginning of what I would one day recognize as the sugar-soaked fatigue in which my youth was lost.

***

After my performance in *The Heiress,* nothing magical happened in school or at home except that my appetite swelled. My dinner helpings enlarged. Snacks multiplied. And I craved sugar.

In school, at the ten-minute break we naively labeled "Nutrition," I ditched Sharon in order to buy a square of whatever cake was available that day through the cafeteria window. Sometimes coming home I'd stop at Cuca's, the little neighborhood store, purchase a jelly donut, shove it into my mouth and slurp it down before I hit the end of the block.

About this time I also started to feel tired a lot. I pushed through it most of the time. But at school we were required to start gym class by a run around the yard. I was always last, lagging about two yards behind everyone else.

But it was my new gastronomic habit that made me nervous. I'd always been thin. "Mother, am I getting fat?"

"No, dear, not at all. What makes you think so?"

She saw my larger meals. I confessed to the donuts and cake. I yearned for her to validate that my food fear was justified. If she did, I might stop. "I ate *two* donuts today." She had to understand how bad it was.

"Oh," she replied, flinging out her invariable denial of my painful experiences, "you won't eat any more donuts."

I won't? Good. I reiterated to myself, *I'm not gaining weight. My eating isn't serious.* I didn't go quite so far as to say, *I won't eat any more donuts.*

One day, ill and home from school, I found myself binging on the previous night's leftovers. Garlic, basil and hot Mexican herbs flavored the tomato sauce, meatballs and beans, lending exquisite taste to Mother's chili. "I'm not getting fat," I intoned aloud, watching myself stand at the sink, eating. "I can stop." But I couldn't stop to heat the dish, let alone sit down with it. By the time I finished, the self-loathing in my chest matched the size of my chili-gorged stomach. I added up the calories and was certain I'd gained five pounds, a whole dress size. I had to stop or I *would* get fat.

And getting fat wouldn't save me from my mother.

I had to do something physically vigorous to burn up those chili calories! But I also had to build real fortifications against Mother in her attack mode, the side of her no one else saw and which, I realized, was what drove me to overeating. The food was great. But I knew I poured savory tastes into my mouth to push Mother out of my mind or, within my mind, to distract myself from her destructive judgments and my self-hatred. What I desperately required instead was a more constructive way to protect myself. What I needed, I decided, was to alter our inflammatory living arrangement. I needed my own room. *Really* my own room.

Tarzan

One afternoon when I was thirteen, I lay on my bed engrossed in the adventures of Tarzan, whose literary version I'd just discovered. My first encounter with the jungle hero had been in his stupid movie characterization. Replaying on television, it obtained only my yawns. But now, astounded by this literary Tarzan's intelligence and absorbed by the epic hero's quest for a lost city, I felt a sudden intrusion into my mind. I looked up. Mother stood in my room, surveying me.

In my mother's house you have to go through the bigger bedroom that was then mine to get to the service porch. Mother always seemed to need to go to the service porch for some reason. Consequently, she was always passing through my room, where she could hardly resist commenting negatively upon its sorry state (it was a disaster) or questioning whether whatever I was doing was what I was supposed to be doing. If I looked too relaxed, her brow wrinkled in concern. I should be struggling more with, well, *something.*

Not that she overtly, or consciously, objected to me enjoying myself. She just felt there must be something else I *should* be doing, because there were always so many unpleasant things to do in life. "You *have to*" do this, she would say. "You *have to*" do that, she would admonish me. "Sometimes you *have to* do things you don't like. You have to *make yourself*, even if you don't *want to."*

Now, on her way to some chore in the service porch, she'd paused, her head tilted to see what I was reading. She frowned and studied me nervously. "Shouldn't you be doing something?"

Typically unable to respond on the moment (for instance, "I *am* doing something"), I answered as a sulky and rebellious teen, "No!"

"What about your homework?"

"I did it." I'd also vacuumed the living room. My lower back ached from dragging the stainless steel canister around and leaning over the hose.

Mother resumed her passage to the service porch with reluctance. I went back to my book. But she continued to traverse my room, each time casting increasingly apprehensive glances in my direction. Without looking up I could almost feel her neurons jumping nervously. I was relaxing, lying around and enjoying my read of Tarzan when I "should be" doing something unpleasant and difficult. That was life.

Ignoring Mother, I continued to read, re-immersing myself in Tarzan's adventure while the early writer part of myself observed how the interweaving threads of the plot wove into a fantastic tale. But my whole body grew steadily more rigid under my mother's repeated passes through my room and her intensifying, bordering-on-hysterical scrutiny as she pursued countless missions in the service porch.

I began to anticipate her reappearances and jerk my head up, shooting angry red sparks at her as if by the sheer power of my glare I could forestall her disapproval, her imminent verbal attack, and erect a battlement between us. But with her every examination of me, her features appeared steadily more strained until at last she looked as if her face would capsize from stress.

I gave up reading and turned on the television. Or I ate. I don't remember. But I never forgot the incident, and on the afternoon I binged on chili three years later, the moment came back to me. As I questioned how I could regain control of my eating, I realized that what I needed was a room of my own.

My own room would provide me with a refuge from my mother's reign of voiced and unvoiced criticisms; her worries and all too vocal cross-examinations of me; her objections to or denial of my every feeling, thought and act; her hysterical outbursts at what she found wrong with me; and the venomous antagonism that was beginning to sear through me in response. Having my own physical room would afford me a parallel interior space of privacy in which I could experience pleasure and not have to defend or account to my mother for it or for anything else. Abruptly, I was certain that having my own room would also demagnetize me from the refrigerator.

As I finished the dishes, soaping off the last unlicked specks of spicy tomato salsa from the chili bowl, I turned my attention toward this objective.

The Goddess

Grunting, sweating and monomaniacal, I lugged mattresses, beds and chests of drawers between our two bedrooms. Shoving and yanking with the strength of a mother lifting a car to save her child, or an obsessive teen trying to work off calories and gain some privacy in the process, I switched the furniture to give myself the petite bedroom and Mother, the relative spaciousness of the larger one. The one connected to the service porch. She could invade herself.

Coming home, she was impressed with my ambition and happy with the new arrangement. I clarified for her, "Now you don't have to go into my room to get to the service porch."

She agreed.

I instructed her, "If you want to come into my room, *please knock."*

"Of course."

Thereafter she gave a perfunctory knock at my bedroom door and, without waiting for my permission, barged in. She felt she had the right.

"Why?" I asked, beside myself. "What gives you the right? This is my room. You *said!*"

"Because what's mine is yours and what's yours is mine," she responded, repeating what she'd often told me, and demolishing the barrier between us that having my own room was meant to erect. Other times she asserted, "I can come in when I want because I AM YOUR MOTHER!" thus calling down the power of the Great Goddess for back-up and unwittingly incorporating into that command her own mother's refrain of divine order: "Mind me, I know best."

With my mother alone, my compulsive smile didn't rule me. I might inwardly creep and skulk in the face of the

Mother Goddess she invoked. But aloud I declared, "I don't care! You can't come in here!"

But she continued to push her way into my room whenever she wanted, stoking my frustration and anger until I was shrieking at the top of my lungs, "Get out!" My rage sprang from a hysterical feeling of helplessness. I'd struggled with all that furniture, hauling my hope with it, and still she invaded my physical space as she did my mind. I still had no privacy anywhere in the house; and now in an already too-small house I was crowded into the smallest room, this tiny hole of a room, like a trapped rat.

New nightmares began.

A gang of killers gets into Mother's house. They are going to kill me. Terrified, I run to the service porch and push out the bottom of the long, large screen that serves as a kind of window. I climb onto the shoulder-high windowsill and roll under the screen, dropping onto the ground outside the house. I tear over the foot or two separating Mother's property from the yard of the next house and take off, running through a strange neighborhood, racing through streets I don't know. My would-be murderers chase me. My *murderers. They are always after* me.

***

For years after I moved out of Mother's house, murderous feelings continued to hunt me down. Through my late teens and twenties I continued to dream of fleeing desperately from the homicidal invaders of Mother's house.

In my thirties, dream apartments replaced Mother's house. Sometimes my dream apartment would be the one in which I actually lived, sometimes not. But in my dreams, my apartment windows or doors don't lock. I can't make them secure. I can't keep the killers out. *I can feel my mattress sinking as a man sits on my bed, holding a knife. I wake in deathly terror, certain someone has really gotten inside and is sitting there.*

As the years proceeded and I went to therapy and worked on my psychological life, I shed a lot of my self-hatred. My dreams reflected that change. But they also dramatized the still unaltered aspects of my psyche. *I've moved into a new apartment, hugely spacious and sunny. But even here, in a "home base" flooded with light, I am unable to lock the doors or windows, I'm afraid of intruders and indeed they come in after me.*

Even after Mother survived her "terminal" cancer and our relationship had deepened into love, the murderers beset me. *I stand on a lovely Japanese bridge in the evening in a cherry blossom garden, and four men in black shoot me. I am at a party having a wonderful time; suddenly, someone knocks me on the head and locks me in the bathroom, plotting to return later and kill me.*

These days there are no killers. Instead, a party of harmless strangers wanders into my apartment. They make themselves at home. I usually can't keep them out or make them leave. I still can't completely control my own psychic space. I still cannot keep other people's attitudes about me, or about anything I perceive or believe, entirely outside my ego boundaries. I take my own position on things. But other people's attitudes and beliefs invade "where I live," and a part of me believes them.

At least my nightmare snakes only rarely return.

Sharon's Secret

Then I was seventeen. High school graduation was only months away. Beyond that day lay college, and escape. If I lasted. Mother and I sat on my bed in my tiny bedroom. Sharon had told me a secret about herself. Mother wanted to hear it.

"I can't tell you," I explained. "It's a secret. She told me in confidence."

"I'm your mother," Mother declared warmly. "You can tell *me*."

"But it's private."

"Tell me. I'm your mother."

"I can't. It's *her* secret!"

"Don't be so selfish!" Her warmth abruptly churned hot with anger. "*Tell me!*"

"I can't!" I pleaded and whined. But her accusations of my selfishness bolted me to guilt. My mind flew back to my first discovery of *that* abominable aspect of my character. It was the one time Mother's bottomless well of pejorative adjectives had foundered.

I'd been five or six when our Sunday routine consisted of my mother sleeping late and then making us pancakes. That Sunday morning she had a nosebleed. She sat at the kitchen table with a blood-soaked rag over her nose. Her nosebleeds were serious. She often had to go to the doctor to stop them. Looking at her, I knew she was uncomfortable. But *I'd* never had a nosebleed and, well, I wanted my pancakes. My mouth watered for pancakes. I could almost taste the maple syrup. I was drooling. I was already a little sugar addict. I said, "But are you going to make pancakes?"

Her head snapped up. Her eyes fixed on me. Her face, partially obscured by the bloody rag, suddenly was ablaze with shock, fury and disgust. "Can't you see I'm having a *nosebleed?* How can you be so—so—so—so—" She grappled for a long moment to pull up her usual flood of qualifiers to annotate the "so" whatever-I-was. But I had *so* appalled her that she finally gave it up and got to the point: *"—so SELFISH???"*

I inched back, mortified. Simultaneously, I rejected that designation. This wasn't right. I was a good person! I knew it! And I was a child. It wasn't fair! But at the same time, deep in my heart, I knew she was right. I was a terrible person. She *loved* me, and look how selfish I was. *I still wanted those pancakes.*

Now, as I kept Sharon's secret, Mother's accusation called back that soul-stunting ignominy. I held out against her but I was wearing down. Then the divine maternal downpour crashed over me. "Tell me," she commanded. "I AM YOUR MOTHER." My resistance washed away into the gutter of my shame, and I broke.

I told her part of Sharon's secret. When I wouldn't divulge the rest, she was beside herself. Why couldn't I just do what she commanded? She was livid. In her mind she had a right to know whatever I knew about Sharon. Like my room, my secrets were my mother's. But how could she make me talk? She'd never struck me so she couldn't start now, although she must have wanted to. Badly.

She reached over and pinched the flesh on my upper arm very hard. "Hey!" *That hurt.* I reached over and pinched her upper arm back. Her eyes widened, surprise infusing her fury. She straightened, surged to her feet and, with an indignant huff, stormed from my room.

I remained sitting on my bed. I slammed my palms over my temples, pressing hard to keep everything inside. My brain seemed to be cracking and flying off into pieces. I had betrayed Sharon and myself by telling Mother *any* of Sharon's secret. Yet I'd betrayed my mother's love by holding back the rest. I'd read R.D. Laing, the Scottish psychiatrist popular at the time. He'd written that in schizophrenia, when the personality cracks, light can come through the fissures. But I didn't see one ray.

Two Mothers

Later, after the conflagration that still lay ahead, Mother would demand the reason for it. "I've loved every moment, every stage of your development!" And of course it was true.

You can see her joy and love in every picture of us when I was an infant, toddler and child, not to mention the series of endearing pet names which she called me from my earliest memory: Little Lamb Chop, Cutie Pie and, more than any other, Little Doll Child. And she really sacrificed a lot for me.

In fact, it's likely that another child or teen would not have responded to my mother as I did. Her overwrought attacks would have rolled off their backs. I have friends who, as children, would just have laughed at my mother's electrically charged commands and denunciations. Most parents damage their children in some way, and Mother was hardly the worst offender. She was never malicious, vicious, competitive or envious of me. She never even spanked me. Her personality simply abraded my specific sensitivities.

Yet perhaps other children might have experienced at least some of my emotional chaos. If a parent only hurts you, then you know how to react. But I had Glenda the Good Witch as well as her sister, the Wicked Witch of the West—or the archetypal Nurturing Mother versus the Devouring Mother.

Or, better yet, Ripley, the Sigourney Weaver character in *Aliens,* versus the alien monster mother. What woman with a raging mother complex can ever forget Ripley, that fantastic super-heroine, buckled into a giant mechanical lifter, its huge metal parts like extensions of her own body as she battles to the death the fanged, double-jawed, drooling monster mother who chases the little girl who has become like Ripley's own daughter? "Mother!" the little girl cries. Ripley advises the monster alien, "Get away from her, *you bitch."* A roar of cheers rose in the theater; my own heart gave Ripley a standing ovation.

But in life the two mothers are the same person. My psyche split accordingly. No matter the zeal with which I fought for the clarity of my own truth, my mother's destructive side was so enmeshed both in her genuine love and self-image of being loving that she totally asphyxiated my perception of reality, which vanished into vapors and murk. Perhaps deep in my bones I battled my mother as madly as I did to try to avoid ending up like my great-aunt, my grandmother's sister, of whom all I ever knew was that she ended up in a mental hospital and probably died there.

***

I graduated high school, made it through summer vacation and left for San Fernando Valley State College. In the Valley, just "over the hill," the college wasn't far from my mother. But it *was* elsewhere. It would be far enough.

Repeating Mother's own history, neither of us thought of my applying for a scholarship. No one we knew, friend or family, mentioned the possibility. I had good grades. I could probably have gotten one. But Mother paid for my first semester without thinking about it.

Classes

Despite switching rooms with Mother, my eating problem had continued. By the end of my last high school semester, I'd gained ten pounds; and the tiredness that had first showed itself with theater candy and started creeping up on me through high school was really taking hold, just in time for college. During my first day in math, a subject in which I usually excelled, I fell asleep at my desk. The only time I'd ever fallen asleep in class before was during high school science classes when the teacher ran a projector next to me and the drone of the machine put me out.

The math teacher whipped out my name. I started, lifting my drowsy head. He told me at the same loud volume, "Get out of this class and don't come back."

I rose shakily. My heart pumped little bursts of humiliation. But after a disoriented moment in the hallway, indignation shot through me. He didn't ask me why I slept. He had no way of knowing if I were sick or what, and had made no attempt to find out. What kind of person was he?

On the other hand, I made sure never to fall asleep in another class.

On the *other* other hand, no other class was that boring.

In fact, my other classes roused an almost unbearable joy.

***

My art teacher, an attractive "young buck," as he called himself, passed out a Renoir print. We waited with pencils poised over our sketchbooks. The teacher instructed us, "Copy the lines and shadows from the print. Don't look at what you're drawing. Just keep your eyes on the picture you're copying from." When I finished, the recognizable representation revived the pleasure I'd felt drawing maps in grammar school. When I got back to the dorm, I sketched my roommate. A few days later I used a magazine picture to draw Marlon Brando. I would keep those sketches pinned to my various walls over the years until the paper dried up and broke into fragments and fell to litter the floor.

After that came my English lit class: *Wuthering Heights, Jane Eyre, Great Expectations.* A woman in her late thirties, the teacher remarked on my affected mannerisms, or perhaps it was my eccentric costume, but not unkindly. My hand constantly up and wagging, down my arm dropped the sleeve of the huge, black, satin, embroidered Cossack-looking shirt Mother had given me (even then, we shared a taste for the exotic) that I wore every day.

My teacher's good-natured patronizing of my apparel didn't faze me. I loved the literary classics I was finally reading. However, my body rebelled at the inundation of sensory detail and genius prose. I didn't know how to process so much great writing. Two well-constructed sentences triggered so many thoughts I lost track of the meaning of both thought and sentence. Moreover, while I loved these books, I had to distill them through my core wrongness, which repelled good experiences. I didn't deserve them.

I fought through these hindrances with, as Mother might have said, "all my might and main."

Then there was my fencing class. My father was a fencing master. I knew nothing about fencing but the idea of learning intrigued me. It would be neat to know an unusual sport. My father had returned from Mexico when I was twelve. He now lived in Phoenix. When I saw him again I could surprise him.

I turned out to be surprised.

***

The story Mother had told me about my father was that, as a young man, he was taking a fencing class and challenged the teacher. When I got to know my father, he laughed. "I waved my foil around, and the teacher ran out the door and never came back."

Whatever really happened, Father took over the class. "I spent my nights reading about fencing and practicing. I had to stay a few steps ahead of my students." It was the greatest mistake of his life. As a professional fencer he could never enter the Olympics. His only choice was to train young fencers to go as his students. That's what he'd been doing in Mexico.

When he'd returned to Los Angeles, he tried for two years to build up students, failed, went to Phoenix where his brother, Bob, lived. He failed there, too, and came back to LA for a year or two before returning again to Phoenix.

I don't actually recall ever attending the college fencing class. But I must have gone once because I know that when the teacher heard my last name, she asked me, "Are you related to—" And she named my father. And I felt his accompaniment. This was the second teacher who knew him. The first had taught in my high school.

***

When my father's mother told me, in our single telephone conversation, that our family had lived in 16th Century Spain, she'd added, "It was during the Inquisition. One of our ancestors was a kind of Clarence Darrow." But theater supplanted law in Father's and my blood. He wanted to be an actor or at least teach fencing to actors, especially the studio stars. Mother told me he didn't get very far. But he did keep a photograph from his youth of himself and Anthony Quinn, and another of himself and Tony Curtis. He also knew "Tony" Quinn in Mexico. Wherever he went throughout his life, my father became involved in local theater, including Los Angeles.

I first discovered this in my high school drama class when a young, two-day, substitute teacher noticed my last name. He asked me, "Are you related to—" He named my father. Because of that, the teacher and I immediately established a special rapport.

But no teacher knew my father in my college theater class, the class that meant the most to me. There I was on my own.

Tim

The theater instructor cast the semester play before I knew anything about it. When I tried out for scenes to be directed by senior students, they yawned at my audition. I instead got the role of hall monitor. I paraded the theater department halls during rehearsals of the class play, telling everyone to be quiet. When not assailing hall talkers (and impressing one student who saw me admonish a teacher for talking), I hung out in the green room, whereupon, after my monitor debut, everyone continued not to notice me.

I was sitting on the green room couch the day a tall, attractive older student with curly brown hair and Irish charm breezed in with a small group. His laughter rolling out, he said to his friends, "No, I'm reading Lawrence Durrell's *The Black Book.* He goes on *for three pages* about Mickey Mouse and his invisible penis."

Everyone joined in his laughter. I gaped. Tim's talent and good looks dazzled me and, as I would discover, most of the young women in the theater department. We thrilled to the songs he wrote and sang, his melodies unforgettable. But most impressive to me, Tim's throwaway lines scattered inklings of a brilliance beneath.

I'd tried to read Durrell's book the previous year but I didn't recall those Mickey Mouse pages. I'd probably spotted them within Durrell's extravagant imagination strung with his lush prose and skipped past them, believing I must have misunderstood. Such originality didn't exist in life. Life was, *You have to do this, you have to do that, even if you don't want to.* Originality meant, *There's something radically wrong with you;* or, *Do, think or say something unusual and People will think you are WEIRD.* For me Mickey and his invisible organ would have appeared incomprehensibly weird.

But Tim possessed the ability to take other people's originality into himself. He trusted and was excited by surprises of genius and responded to them spontaneously. He bore no fear of his spontaneity or what it might reveal about him. Just the opposite. Tim astounded me. The new thing, the unknown thing, the elaborate and fantastic thing, added to rather than threatened him; it enabled him to further explore his originality and enjoy his life. He made Durrell's book part of himself.

It strikes me this quality also drew me to Don. However different his style was from Tim's, Don was an original and incorporated his originality into his life. I saw this after one of the discussions he often held with his audience following the plays he directed for the LAAT. During one such discussion, someone in the audience brought to Don's attention an unusual fact missing from the play. Don said, "Oh, I wish I'd known that." He laughed, turning to Guy. "You know how much mileage I get out of an exotic piece of information." Guy laughed. Don not only enjoyed his own eccentricities, he made them work for him. Other People enjoyed his weirdness. He was unique *and it was good.* Don had personified the possibility that I might one day enjoy my own uniqueness.

And now here was Tim, exemplifying the same possibility along with a breezy freedom that I'd never seen in anyone. I became friends with another young woman who shared my crush on Tim. Together we got ourselves invited to parties at his apartment. There he kept a life-size cardboard cutout of Nancy Wilson, who substituted in his heart for an unnamed, beautiful Black woman with whom he was in love but who was married. Tim pointed to the multi-hued pixels of Nancy Wilson and said, "She's colored." I thought this was hilariously witty. I was certain that the woman with whom Tim, this amazing guy, was in love, must really be something. Who was she? What was she like? I never dreamed for one second that, in another time and place, when Tim remained only a flashy memory, this woman and I would become the closest of friends while, for three decades, we remained unaware of this previous link between us.

Yet even as joy scintillated in my veins whenever Tim was around, exuding his gems of originality, a nebulous depression also began to settle over me. In the end what really electrified me about Tim was his fearless exultation in life itself, which, in my deeper self, I rejected. I was attracted to Tim because he loved life in a way I could not. He personified my own potential, but it seemed reachable only when I was in his presence.

Of course, there was the further depressing element of having a crush on someone and knowing he wasn't remotely interested in me. I was not yet eighteen, I'd never had a boyfriend, and I longed for love. Fantasies of romance, culled from movies and enhanced by hormones, danced in my heart like Sugar Plum Fairies. Only one thing was worse than knowing that a man I liked would never find me attractive: when I thought and dreamed a man I liked *could* be drawn to me, and it didn't happen. The biggest such event was about to occur.

***

Each year when I was a child, I thought for some reason that my father might come back from Mexico at Christmas. I told other kids importantly, "This Christmas MY FATHER is going to visit me." They looked at me askance, as if to say, "Okay? Yeah? So?" Their expressions indicated they thought I was a little crazy. But they didn't care one way or another. And Father never came.

Now my father invited me to visit him in Phoenix for Christmas vacation. He sent me money for the visit. I'd never received any gift from him that I could remember. The bus money was evidence of the love I'd always known he felt.

That trip would direct the next vast swath of my life.

The Sign

I sat looking out the bus window as the Greyhound rolled into the city. Neon signs lined the night streets. Among them there rose up, upon a tall building, one that read, BANK OF PHOENIX. I stared at it. Exhilarated and stunned, I discovered myself thinking, *Phoenix isn't just a television image. It really exists. Other places exist outside of my mother's fixation on me!* I didn't have this feeling about college. It wasn't far enough after all. Until that moment, I'd glimpsed reality outside my mother's web only in a few rarefied instances. One had occurred when I was around eight, on the day I almost died.

Mother frequently took me to the beach. She loved to body surf, gliding in on the foamy waves. One day I was playing by myself near the shore. I hadn't gone into the water very far when a wave knocked me over. The undertow snatched my feet from under me. My feet scrambled frantically as the water flipped me over and over, but I couldn't find land. In a panic I tried to scream but only swallowed more seawater. The salt stung the back of my throat and plugged and burned my nose. I couldn't breathe. My arms wheeled furiously as I tumbled. No one noticed my distress. Where was my mother, who was always into everything in my life? I was going to die! Terror bore through me in fierce concert with the ceaseless waves. No one came to save me.

When the sea finally released me, I staggered up the damp shore and over the hot dry sand, exhausted from fright and weighted down with salt water, sand and the world of gravity to which I'd returned. I found Mother sitting on her towel, chatting with her best friend, Alta. I'd nearly drowned, or felt I had. But as I approached my mother, I could see she was completely unaware of my trauma. Nor did she sense or see in me anything unusual when I stopped before her. She simply looked up at me and smiled. "Hello, honey. Are you having a good time?"

With a jolt of shocked disappointment and relief, I realized that nearly drowning had severed me from her obsessive love. I'd had a completely private moment. The incident implanted itself deep within me. Through death I could escape her control, her perception of me and, with it, my own belief in my wrongness.

Movies provided another of my escapes. Identifying with the gorgeous and charismatic actors as well as the singular characters they portrayed, I experienced my own individuality as a thing of fantastic energy and creativity; that is, as a good thing, not weird or wrong. But once the movie ended, I snapped back into my mother's image of me and of what she needed me to be, and of what I needed to be to retain her love. Once more she alone knew what I felt, needed, believed, thought, saw. I was less than nothing. I was a failure.

I had learned I could also escape her, and discover who I was, if I became an actress myself.

After that, one last path to myself remained: what I thought of as love. Whenever I had a crush on an attractive guy like Tim, I flew into such a whirlwind of hormones and dreams that the intensity alone took me out of my mental prison. If I ever found a loving relationship with a guy, I believed I'd also begin to live from my true and original self. And, again, I would know that self was good.

But now this sign, BANK OF PHOENIX, presented further possibility. It revealed that other geographies actually existed. Then why couldn't I be different in them than I'd been taught to be or had imagined myself to be where my surroundings were familiar?

And then there was a man: For the first and only time in my life, I saw an exciting, attractive man, centered myself in an intuitive link with him, and emitted a sympathetic vibration.

Nick Nolte

Had that sign, BANK OF PHOENIX, freed me from my normal self-image? Or was it my father inviting me to visit him and sending money for the trip, a previously unheard-of phenomenon? Was it my father actually *being there for me* in his love, and at Christmas, of all times, the season that since my childhood I'd fantasized that *he* would visit *me*?

In any case, in Phoenix as elsewhere, Father belonged to the local theater group. After picking me up at the bus stop and leaving my (physical) baggage in his apartment, he took me to a cast party. I was slender; during my first months at college I'd lost all but a few pounds of my recent excess; and now the party buoyed me up. An unusual energy was buzzing through me when, off in one room, I observed a tall, blond, handsome, charismatic guy. With an anomalous self-confidence never to be repeated, I thought, *I'm going to meet him.*

I'd once asked Sharon, "How do you flirt?" Guys all swarmed around her.

"I don't know." She shrugged. "I just kind of feel a bubbly sensation."

"Bubbly?"

"I kind of...*effervesce.*"

I never effervesced.

But half-an-hour later the attractive guy and I were squeezing past each other in a doorway of the crowded party amid the overlapping loud conversations and louder music. Both of us swimming through the bright colors, cigarette smoke and whirling fumes of alcohol infusing the air, we smiled at each other, our smiles taking in the ambience.

I effervesced.

We started talking, went into the living room, sat on the couch and talked for two hours. His eyes were watery as he told me something sad. My own eyes went starry. *Oh,* I thought, *he's so sensitive!* Actually, he was a little drunk.

But smart. Really smart. And I felt we had so much in common that something might really happen. From the party he took me to his parents' house. They weren't home. We went into a bedroom and made out for a long time, kissing and kissing. (Make love, not war, was my sixties political credo, but personally I planned virginity until marriage.) Afterwards, he poured me champagne. I was ecstatic. I was *different* with him. I was different this night! My new life lay ahead. I had spoken to an attractive, talented actor without inhibition, without The Smile, and now I was drinking the first champagne of my life with him.

His name was Nick Nolte. An aspiring actor, he was playing Prince Charming in the local children's production of *Cinderella*. The following afternoon my father dropped me off at the theater to see Nick's performance. Nick took the stage with charm (he was, after all, Prince Charming). He was magnetic despite his hangover.

Backstage afterwards he kind of remembered me. Pushing his fingers back through his blond hair, he asked me whether he looked bloated. "A little," I replied, uncomfortable at confirming something negative about him. He was nice but I saw that his interest in me had been transient. I became my familiar self again.

He offered to drive me back to my father's apartment. On the way, Nick's sporty white convertible hurtling along the otherwise empty highway, he told me a story I'd never forget. It made me hope again. I was sure we shared a similar spirit.

"This guy I know," Nick said, the desert spread around us, our faces cooking under the powerful sun despite a brisk temperature, "Billy. He was in a card game with another guy in a cabin. Billy was pressuring the other guy to do something. The other guy said no. Once. Billy kept pushing. The other guy didn't say anything else. He just sat there playing cards. A spider crossed the table in front of them. The guy picked the spider up, put it in his mouth and swallowed it. And just kept playing."

"Wow." I gasped. We sat a moment in silence, thinking about the nonverbal genius of spider-eater's resistance to pressure. I said, "I could see Marlon Brando doing something like that."

"Yeah." Nick looked almost shaken by the story. I don't think he particularly wanted to share an interesting tale with me. He didn't know me. But he was in the grip of this mental tableau and it just came up naturally in the context of our conversation, which was about acting.

I was telling him about Don, Guy and the LAAT. Nick's story reminded me of a movie scene which displayed similar brilliance. The scene occurred in a samurai movie that had comprised one of the LAAT field trips.

In the movie the bad guys break into Toshiro Mifune's room, swords raised to kill him. He glances up calmly from his dinner, snaps the points of his chopsticks together and catches a fly circling the bowl of rice in his lap. The bad guys gape, mutter, grunt and fall all over each other getting out of the room. If Mifune's that fast with his chopsticks, he'd slaughter them in a fight. Once they're gone, Mifune as calmly releases the fly and continues eating.

This scene passed through my mind as cool air gusted over our hair in the bright afternoon. Then I recalled something I'd learned at the LAAT itself. I read Freidrich Durrenmatt's *The Visit* when Don assigned it. Yet, as usual, I'd missed its ingenious theatricality until Don articulated it.

"A woman returns to the town where she became pregnant by her lover when she was young," said Don. "The town kicked her out. Her own people punished her while permitting her lover to achieve prominence in the town. But she married and became immensely wealthy, and now she returns to her hometown as a widow. She says she'll give the town a million dollars if they'll execute the man who impregnated her.

"The people act insulted," Don reminded us. "They're indignant. They won't sell out their friend for all the money in the world. But the woman stays in the town. She knows her people. No one acknowledges accepting her offer. No one takes a penny. But you see people start walking around in new shoes."

Such dramatic subtlety had stupefied me—that artists thought like this. Creativity like this existed! And now Nick was sharing an incident from real life that exhibited the same genius of physicalizing an inner, unspoken truth. Nick's general attitude was loose, open, but an intensity underlay it; and he spoke of this event as if it held a secret he couldn't quite grasp. I understood that and desperately wanted to share with him the samurai scene and the story of the shoes. He'd appreciate those theatrical parallels with real life. He would appreciate *me* for recognizing them. He might like me.

But the possibility of communicating so important a part of myself to someone as important to me as he was, paralyzed me. Even as my imbecilic smile returned, the samurai movie and Don's insight about *The Visit* swam slowly past my mind like tropical fish in iridescent colors; while I, in a kind of daze, helplessly locked into myself, just watched the fish and the moment come and go. I'd gotten out the sentence about Brando. That was the most I could accomplish.

Afterwards, I tormented myself. Would I have made an impression on Nick had I spoken? Would we have connected? Probably not. My need for love was so neurotic; and in any case, Nick was set on a particular course, with needs and drives and an emotional coherence completely alien to my life. Maybe he wasn't even thinking about the theatricality of the spider eater. Maybe the sheer macho cool of the event was what captivated him.

But had I spoken, at least I'd have been myself. That was always the most painful thing. I betrayed myself with my silence and stupid smile and never knew what would have happened if I'd dared reveal myself.

I did, however, break out of my incarcerating psychical walls one more time. Just before we left the desert and hit the city streets, I saw standing alone in the distance a stone outcropping. Right out of numerous Westerns and a few science fiction movies I'd loved, the outcropping unveiled a geographical reality, *another place* that, in this case, with a thrill of wildness, I felt manifested in the outer world my interior drive for originality. The excitement of adventure swept through me at the sight of it. I pushed myself up on the car seat and I waved at that fantastic giant rust-red tooth of the desert. "Goodbye, Phoenix!" I called.

Nick shot me a look. "Why did you do that?"

No one had ever asked me, with genuine curiosity, why I'd done a particular spontaneous thing. "I don't know. I just felt like it."

Nick digested this. He stored spontaneous moments. They fueled his acting juices. Through most of my life, starting with Nick and Tim, I've had crushes on men who lived out that kind of passion, just as I've been strongly attracted to men who were not there for me.

I spent the rest of the week with my father.

I would run into Nick a year later at the Raincheck, a famous Hollywood watering hole for actors. He didn't remember me until I mentioned Don, Guy and the LAAT. Then he said, "Oh, yeah." Nick appeared in his star-making role in a television mini-series the following year.

It had never occurred to either of us to question why I'd said, "Good-bye, Phoenix," instead of, "Hello."

Father

I'd always carried the image of my father as carefree. Although he went to Mexico when I was so young, and I rarely saw him after he came back to Los Angeles, I always felt, or fantasized, that had he been around while I was growing up, he would have acted as a buffer against my mother, in his style as well as his presence. This visit showed him to be just as I imagined.

The previous night, after the cast party and my kissing adventure with Nick, I returned around midnight to my father's apartment. He voiced no criticism about my arrival at the late hour, nor did he question me. He seemed a little hurt that I would have another interest taking up my time while I visited him. But he was thoroughly nonjudgmental, unhorrified, unterrified and unhysterical. He gave me what I so urgently craved at my mother's house: my own space.

He was my favorite parent.

Of course, while I regarded him as lighthearted, Mother had considered him irresponsible. For one thing, there was his gambling. Mother told me recently that he'd stop in Gardena and burn up his salary. "He was always late. Sometimes he didn't get home until midnight. I was terrified about what might have happened to him. I knew it was time to get a divorce the night he didn't come home and I wasn't worried any more. I was angry."

Whenever I'd spoken about his easy-going ways, Mother reminded me of the time he took me to the beach. Either I was two and it was just before he left for Mexico, or I was twelve and he'd first arrived back in LA "He forgot your sweater!" Mother exhaled in shock and horror. I thought, *Who cares?* All I recall is being happy to go anywhere with him. I wasn't cold.

He showed his care in areas that, to me, counted more. He took me to Tijuana to see the bullfights and made sure we left as soon as the clowns finished leaping over and dancing around the bulls. I never saw a drop of blood. For years afterwards I remained unaware that matadors torment and kill the bull.

The only time I'd see a different side of Father would be in the future when I started taking fencing lessons from him. As he showed me how to hold my foil or place my feet, he announced in a disgusted tone, "No, no, no, no, no, no. Not like *that.*" He verbally clobbered all his students with the same demeaning tone. Startled and demoralized to see this negative side of him, I would only take a few lessons. But no hint of that side of him appeared during my college Christmas visit.

I found him charming and mentally cast him in a movie. His apartment was overrun with roaches. As he made eggs for us the first morning, a critter skittered toward his foot. He lifted his foot courteously to let it pass beneath. "Oh, hello," he said. I pictured Dean Martin playing him in a movie. Very suave. (I bought bug spray and saturated every inch of his living quarters. Dead roaches appeared on the floor, in cupboards and others crawled into my bed to die. Years later I would wonder if I'd contributed to the cancer that killed my father.)

Returning to college after my vacation, some core strength in my emotional center fell apart.

I rarely seem to have been aware, when major events occurred in my life, of their true cause.

Breakdown

Back in the college theater department, I won no acting roles in student scenes or roused any interest whatsoever from Tim. My food cravings reanimated themselves like movie monsters even as my fatigue achieved complete power over my life. I stumbled from my dorm bed and trundled off to the cafeteria where, as in my childhood, my drooling proclivities seized upon donuts. I gobbled them powdered, jellied, plain, glazed. Then I retreated to my dorm room and slept as if in a coma. Within weeks, I gained fifteen pounds and could hardly get up except to hit the cafeteria for more donuts.

I quit going to classes. I lay in bed reading classics. I luxuriated in *Great Expectations,* which I could enjoy with no one anxiously questioning whether I should be doing something else. But soon I could no longer bear to take into myself that joy.

I sank into depression as if into a dark, too soft, too low couch, like one of my mother's couches, from which you could not pull yourself up without slipping a disc. I didn't think the depression would ever end. This would have frightened me except that the only thing I cared about any more was that I didn't care about anything.

The BANK OF PHOENIX sign had shocked me into a new awareness. Other realities existed in the world than the one I knew. The *world* existed, not just my narrow experience of it; and in the different places of that larger outer reality, my inner reality could also change. Yet I'd come back to college as invisible as when I left; just as before, no male person that I liked, liked me; and why should they, now, any more than before? I was attracted to guys who shone. They possessed a passion for life I myself lacked, perhaps had never felt. They possessed a self-confidence that I hungered to feel so I tried to live vicariously, through them. Moreover, as soon as I approached someone I wanted to impress, I compulsively inhibited myself from saying what I really thought or felt, which might have been interesting to them and at least would have been genuine. Instead, I offered only The Smile, and appeared foolish, ignorant and mediocre. That is what my trip ultimately revealed, and it literally sickened me. I'd been to Phoenix but inside my head I hadn't gone anywhere. Nothing had changed. There was no Greyhound bus to a different self.

I didn't care about my school record any more than anything else. But I did calculate that if I should ever care again, and wanted to return to school, I should protect my future self. I talked to all my teachers. I told them about my depression and that I'd just come back from a visit with my father. I let the obvious psychological implications hang in the air. I didn't think they would accept the reasons I actually believed responsible (Tim, Nick, the sign) for what was called my "nervous breakdown." My teachers accepted the father story and marked my class grades as "incomplete" instead of "failed." I thought I was so clever.

But the truth was that such close quarters with my father had, without my being aware of it, elicited for me our previous relationship: his decade-long absence in Mexico, his many departures from LA to Phoenix once he'd returned, and all my emotions surrounding these events.

Indeed, I wonder how unconscious I must have been to miss seeing his role in the depression that sent me back to my mother. My least favorite parent.

Faux Father

One day at age twelve, I was sick and home from school. Eating lunch and watching my favorite daytime program, *Crusader Rabbit with Sheriff John*, I picked up the ringing telephone. The man who was calling asked if I was Alexa. I said yes. He said, "I'm your father."

My heart started pumping out anger and fear. How could someone be that mean? "I don't believe you." I was *terrified* of believing him. Sheriff John and the Rabbit shut themselves off from my awareness. No scrap of memory came to me about another man on the phone when I was around three, who also said he was my father.

In that earlier conversation, Mother and I had been eating dinner. When the phone rang, Mother picked it up, talked a moment, then handed me the receiver. "Here's your father."

I took the phone, starting to cry. My father had gone away. He'd been gone a long time. He had not contacted me and I missed him horribly. The man on the phone said soothing words. "I love you," he said. But something was wrong. As he spoke, my tears dried up. He said, "I can't come see you right now but I love you." But I was confused. I didn't disbelieve him because my mother had handed me the phone. She knew who he was! I must be wrong. *But he didn't feel like my father.* Did I not know my own father, whom I loved so much? *Was I crazy?*

When I hung up, Mother asked if I felt better. I told her what she obviously expected and wanted to hear. "Yes." But I felt hollow, as if my love and grief had been stolen and my body were separate from me. My self-trust was gone. With it went my self.

Somehow the incident came up a few years ago. Mother told me, "You were so upset after your father left, I had to do something. You were crying all the time. When you heard wind on the porch at night, you'd sit up in bed and say, 'I think I hear my father coming.'" So she'd asked a male friend to pose as my father. "I thought it would make you feel better."

I chose not to inform her that her attempt to ease my pain had caused me to lose grounding and confidence in my ability to deal with reality. I didn't explain how the experience had taken something from my soul, making me lonelier than ever. If I'd spoken, Mother would have interpreted my words as an accusation, and I might have meant them as such, and there was no point bringing back the past when our new relationship was so good.

But when my father called, when I was twelve and he'd just come back from Mexico, I plunged into a whirlwind of confusion. The moment he told me who he was, tears brimmed in my eyes then stormed down my face. No recollection came to me of the earlier telephone conversation with my faux father. But he lingered in my unconscious and now he undermined me. This time I felt I *was* talking to my father. But I feared to trust my senses and face the pain and disappointment if I were wrong. Yet he seemed sincere. *He seemed like my father.* Why should someone try to fool me? But why should I believe a stranger on the phone? And if this was really my father, what was he doing here, anyway? My father was a phantom in Mexico, who loved me, but never showed it.

***

Also with the best of intentions, Mother lied on another Father-related matter throughout my childhood. She told me she was sending Father all my report cards, my good grades, my maps and the other pictures I drew; and she told him about the stories I wrote. All that time I pictured Father receiving these scraps of myself, keeping up with my efforts and talents through the years. I could almost see him holding them, although he never called; and he wrote to me only once during his ten-year absence.

That letter contained just a few sentences scribbled on textured notepad paper, telling me he'd gotten married. Along with his letter came a photograph of his Mexican wife. She was, one of his friends from Mexico would tell me years later, "one of the most beautiful women in Mexico."

I must not have told my mother about the letter, or else she forgot. Either way, she recently informed me in disgust, "I didn't know where he was. He never told me. He never called. He never wrote. The whole time he was in Mexico I never knew if he was dead or alive."

Hearing this admission decades after my father's death, I felt as if my heart fell over inside me. *You never knew? But you told me you mailed all my schoolwork and everything to him!* All the time Father was in Mexico I thought he knew these things about me—and just didn't bother to write. He loved me. I knew this. I never doubted his love. But I wasn't worth the effort of his writing to me. I could be loved, but never enough for him to make an effort to respond to my school efforts, to be there for me.

Yet what would have been different had I possessed the truth? Even if Mother did know where he was and really sent him my things, would he have written? He could have written or called without that impetus. The fact that he called when he returned to LA showed he had my number. And he knew where I lived.

Yet I would never feel angry at him. My emotions were unreasonable and unjust. But, until Mother's and my reconciliation, my anger flew at her like screaming ravens for what she did, rather than at him for what he didn't do.

***

I gripped the phone. Crusader Rabbit receded to a meaningless babble. Was the man at the other end of the line really my father, as he claimed? I wept.

"I'll come over tomorrow," he promised.

"But how do I know you're my father?"

He repeated that he was. The more convinced I let myself become, the harder I cried. I cried so hard that he decided, "I'll come over right now." When he arrived, I raced to open the door. I clung to him, hugging him, my tears gushing. But we were not alone.

At that time Mother kept her bed in the living room, gave me the big bedroom and, in the small one, installed the consecutive women she hired to take care of me while she worked and went to night school. Mrs. Mason was my current sitter. A big-boned, sentimental old woman, she lumbered into the living room to watch the reunion. But my emotional display in her presence embarrassed my father. He put his hands on my shoulders and kind of moved me away from him while, flushed with embarrassment, he smiled and shrugged at Mrs. Mason.

Even with my father, my deepest feelings, expressed with spontaneity, revealed my wrongness. I embarrassed him. Mrs. Mason was more important to him than I was.

I smiled to show I was okay with him moving me back from him. I was afraid my humiliating tears would drive him away. I forced myself to stop crying. But, doing so, I jumped into my head, leaving my body feeling disconnected from me. An emotional unreality set in. *Smile or your father won't like you.* The only feelings of which I remained aware were love and a desperation that he not leave me.

I knew about his gambling (although not that this was the reason Mother divorced him), and I loved to play cards. I played obsessively with neighborhood kids and usually won. I asked Father, "Do you want to play gin rummy?"

"All right." I sensed he held little interest in the game but he wanted to do something with me.

I won. After that game, I lost all interest in playing cards or any kind of game, ever again.

A handful of years later, halfway through my first college semester and after my visit to my father, my favorite parent, I lost interest in everything. I left college and moved back in with Mother.

Gandhi

Don had not only blasted open my mind with his insights into acting and theater, and with the way he turned his eccentricities into benefits. He also shared his personal politics in class. What I learned of them would become a crucial element in the demented fury building inside me in my mother's house.

I wasn't apolitical. From my earliest years Mother took me to peace demonstrations and ban-the-bomb marches, never once missed voting (Democratic); and for decades after Stalin's massacres were revealed, she clung to the USSR as the Communist dream that lived in her own generous heart. But Don was the first person I ever knew who talked about Gandhi and nonviolence and, due to direct experience, I immediately got what he said.

When I was thirteen, I discovered a cruel streak in myself. Junior High gym class began with everyone forming lines. Each girl put her hand on the shoulder of the girl in front of her to create the proper distance. I pushed down extremely hard on the shoulder of the girl in front of me, deliberately hurting her. Yet Sharon forgave me and became one of my closest lifelong friends. I did something equally mean to Gita, another girl; I don't recall what. Then one day in a class we shared I was so ill I practically passed out. Gita asked me with genuine concern if I was okay and then called over the teacher. "Alexa is sick!" Feverish, dizzy and weak, I thanked Gita, overcome with gratitude for her help and shame at the way I'd treated her in the past, for no reason.

"Gandhi called his nonviolent movement *Satyagraha,*" Don explained. "It's a Sanskrit word that translates simultaneously as Truth Force, Soul Force and Love Force. Gandhi tells us that violence doesn't stop violence. Violence creates more violence. But love does stop it because love is the soul and truth of our being."

Kindness and forgiveness from those two girls had stopped my violence toward them and transformed Sharon into a lifelong friend. Don's discussions put my personal experiences in a political context. Listening to his commentaries on nonviolent political action from my sixteenth year onward, I increasingly wanted to explore the subject. Gandhi said something like, "If love be not the core of man's being, then the whole of my argument falls to pieces." I could feel in these words a balm for my own seared soul and lost truths. I thought at times about a career that included writing as well as acting. I intended to write tales that illuminated Satyagraha. I was certain I could find ways to dramatize it in exciting, entertaining, probably science fiction action-adventures.

When I left college midway through my first semester, I lacked the drive to return to Don's theater. Fatigue, depression and apathy owned me. If I cared about anything it was this potential future, as a teller of Satyagraha tales. Vague plots of nonviolent yet heroic magnitude began to coruscate in my imagination. The desire to write them was germinating deep inside me. And these potential stories that I harbored, these future Gandhian epics, however indefinite and undeveloped at the moment, told me who I was, and this was a knowledge which, more dreadfully than ever, I needed to possess. For the conflict between Mother and me was scaling toward all-out warfare.

Home Again

I was eighteen and Mother still barged into my tiny room. It was her house and, she let me know, she had the right. Her dissertations on my shortcomings persisted in hysterical outbursts, and nightmares consumed my sleep. I couldn't stop eating. A size fourteen, I was getting fatter. My mother controlled my physical space, and I couldn't control my psychic space. Every time she found and, invariably voiced, something wrong with me, I lived more deeply in my wrongness than the moment before, no matter how angrily I rebelled against her.

I had to get a job so I could leave. I started working downtown for the government as a typist. But fatigue ached in my veins. In the huge beehive office, a cacophony of typewriters clacking away around me, I kept leaning over my own typewriter, unable to maintain a vertical posture or even catch my breath. I forced myself back up but...what was I just typing? Physical weakness was compounded by mental drag.

Two weeks after I began the job, I quit. I just couldn't do it.

Then what lay ahead? My mother. Her house. Her rules and intrusions. My eternal wrongness, fused into my genes, my soul, and no episode of it ever missed. Every fiber of my body screamed, I CAN'T LIVE LIKE THIS! But I saw no alternative, and none, or nothing sane, presented itself. If I couldn't work, I couldn't get out.

We would never afterwards speak directly of the incident with the knife that was about to occur. Now that event belongs to another life, to two other people; except when I come here, to my mother's house, and from our past, even that long distant past we shared, the incident comes again to life like the ominous flare of a solar storm reaching across the light-years from a distant star.

Possessed

Healthy family life traditionally revolves around sharing meals. In my family of two, with my uncontrollable eating, meals became the point of greatest hostility between Mother and me. All day I binged. I craved bread, ate a half a loaf of peanut butter sandwiches, went to the local grocery store and bought a cake. Then I gorged on all the protein leftovers I could find in the refrigerator, cold chicken, fish, lamb chops. When Mother came home at night, she demanded I sit and eat dinner with her.

"I can't," I'd beg her.

"Just sit down and have a few bites!" She'd worked so hard all week, all my life, and put further effort, her last ounce of strength, into making a delicious meal *for me.*

"But I ate all day."

But she didn't care.

On the night our battles came to a head, spaghetti sauce burbled on the stove, its tomatoey scent wafting about the kitchen and living room. Cooking separately, meatballs sizzled, and noodles in their colander signaled, *Come hither.* As usual, Mother insisted I join her. I told her I just couldn't. My loss of control had never been as bad as that day. "I've already eaten enough for a week!" I argued, gripped by self-hatred. I'd counted and obsessed over every wretched calorie. "If I sit down with you, I won't be able to stop."

"The least you can do is act companionable," Mother replied with scorn and anger.

"Just let me go into my room while you eat!"

"Don't be so selfish!"

Selfish—again! Shame twisted my entrails. Crucified by my selfishness! I remembered Mother's nosebleed and those pancakes I craved so long ago, the craving for which had first, and indelibly, marked me as selfish. And now here it was again, only in reverse: Mother was a fabulous cook.

The one thing I could do to save myself from further uncontrollable gluttony and hateful fat was avoid her mouth-wateringly wonderful food. But now I was selfish for wanting to *not* eat her food with her.

My insides seethed with my incorrigible ingratitude even as I hated her for making me feel this shame.

I sat down with her. How could I not? I had to redeem myself.

I took a few bites. Just as I'd feared, once I started eating, I couldn't stop. "I told you!" I accused her, finishing up my third plate.

"You don't have to eat all that," she countered, reason well on her side, which only made me angrier, and hungrier. I forked up more pasta and spooned more sauce over it. I ate until every noodle, meatball and drop of Italian-spiced spaghetti sauce was gone. Then it was time to do the dishes, to stand, by force of will against my overwhelming fatigue. My every cell felt weighted by a ball and chain. But it was time to do the dishes—just exactly the way my mother wanted them done.

Doing the dishes was my chore in any meal-making. But everything had to be exactly right. But I could never do *anything* quite right, including my housework activities.

I cleared the table. My stomach about to blow up from dinner and my head about to explode from the feverish convulsion of my emotions, I didn't think I could stand another moment of myself, my mother or my life.

The Knife

"Oh, that's very nice, dear, but *that over* ***there...*"** Mother's energy without fail disregarded my efforts in favor of my mistakes despite her own imperfect housekeeping. When she herself dusted, she made wide, blind, whooshing sweeps of the dust cloth which left upon the furniture surface clean but indiscriminate roads through the dusty overlay. But when *I* cleaned, not only could I leave no speck of dust. I also had to replace each knick-knack in precisely the right place. If I was off by one nanometer, whether by error or an attempt to bring my creativity to bear by slightly rearranging her knick-knacks, that nanometer of alteration became the sole focus of the full force of her critical attention.

Washing dishes proved no different. "Over there, dear. You missed that spot," she'd inform me, as she did this night, pointing to a small red blotch of spaghetti sauce at the edge of the sink. I stared at it. A furnace of rage blazed up in my chest. My forehead burned. I hadn't even finished the dishes. It wasn't fair! I thought. *I'd have seen that spot!*

Or maybe not. Suddenly, I didn't care. I felt myself revolt. I reviled myself and I detested my mother. *Don't be selfish.* I was going insane.

I failed her. She failed me. *I was a failure.* She dismissed me as inconsequential or attacked me as an object of her horror and terror. She praised my creative endeavors but only because she liked her own creativity, and when I was creative, I was a positive reflection of her, Mother's "Little Doll Child;" her little doll, not a human girl. But when I did something that reflected a part of herself she disliked or feared, there was something *radically wrong* with me. My instincts and emotions, thoughts and dreams, didn't exist unless they pleased her, and if they did exist despite her displeasure, they exposed this wrongness of mine which comprised my innermost self and existed in everything from the way I walked to my fingernails to the snot in my nose.

I'd once tried to explain to Sharon how I felt about myself. I'd looked inside myself and described the picture I saw. "It's like I'm stabbing my heart over and over and over forever in furious self-hate."

"How awful," Sharon said.

"And it's happening all the time. Sometimes I hate myself more and stab harder. I can't stop the feeling."

Now I paused over the soapy water and dishes. A wet sponge in one hand, I held in the other the carving knife I'd been sponging clean. Now I held a real knife.

Suddenly gone was any understanding I bore toward Mother for *her* emotional burdens. Our family history had instilled in her a profound insecurity with which she was not equipped to deal. But suddenly my empathy for her was obliterated. Instead, every negative thing she'd ever said to me, and about me to others, congealed and transmogrified in my depths. I just couldn't do anything good enough for her! I just couldn't get it right!

And I'd never get out.

I was stuck in my mother's house, unable to work, a prisoner of my fatigue, and equally unable to break free from my own paralyzing neuroses that locked me outside of any self-trust, self-confidence or self-love. I smiled compulsively to compensate for my wrongness and seethed with hatred toward myself for that smile. I punished myself by binging and soothed myself by binging more and could halt neither behavior.

Yes, she loved me so much, I was her reason for living, she thought about me all the time; but that was too much for me to carry. And at the same time, I was her reflection and her appendage, and that was too little. Either way, never once in my life had I felt that my mother saw or treated me with respect as an individual separate from her, with my own soul and integrity, and so I never felt that I possessed either.

You missed that spot. Dear.

I wasn't smiling now. I turned toward Mother. Gripping the warm sudsy handle of the long knife, sweat slick on my face from the kitchen heat and my own inner blaze, I backed her to the yellow kitchen wall, placed the blade point against her stomach and imagined it going into her flesh. I foresaw hot blood pouring out.

Denial and fear clashed in her features. I could see she shared the same nightmarish image.

She couldn't believe it. It was ghastly. *This isn't happening,* her expression insisted. But her eyes flicked back and forth between the knife and my face. I could almost hear her bowels roil with the fright that froze her to the spot just as I, knife in hand, was paralyzed by my helpless fury and hate.

I gripped the handle tighter, consumed by my lurid compulsion. I'd never get escape while she was alive. I'd be under her ever-condemning thumb for the rest of my life and I would continue to believe her assessment of me, despite myself. How I ached to plunge in the knife and stop my torment. Killing her was the only way to unshackle myself from her power.

Mother flattened herself harder into the wall to evade the knifepoint, which I held an inch away from her. The refrigerator crowded her to one side. The hallway entrance rose up on the other. But if she tried to slip sideways into the hallway, the slightest turn would run her into the knife. Instinct also warned her that the least movement would ignite my insanity to the final act. As her terrified gaze shot back to my face, she didn't fight or say a word. Instead, on her countenance a patina of bewilderment appeared over her terror. How, when, had our relationship, which she'd always deemed perfect—or at least she'd thus deemed her role in it—turned into *this?*

And what did I plan to do?

Yes, what? Suddenly that was my question, too. I hesitated. A furious, hot roaring filled my head. A single, seemingly lucid thought crossed my mind. I thought,

Gandhi. I thought: *If I kill my mother, no one is going to believe me when I write stories about nonviolence.*

I saw myself writing these stories from prison. I wasn't afraid of prison. My mother wouldn't be there. But what point would there be if people ridiculed my stories as the ravings of a madwoman? No one would understand why I'd killed her. No one would see anything more of our relationship than any of her friends did. She was the Perfect Mother, and I, already viewed as spoiled, would become the Bad Seed.

There was no way around this truth and, therefore, no escape in this direction. I took a step back from my mother. I watched her steal instantly around the kitchen doorway and scurry down the short, narrow hallway to her bedroom, the larger of the two. I returned to the sink and finished washing the dishes.

Boundaries

For years afterwards I thought I'd stopped myself because of my nonviolent ideals and dreams of writing epic adventures of nonviolence. Only recently have I realized my true impetus. For all the psychological boundaries Mother crossed, she had never physically struck me. "I made that decision before you were born," she told me recently. "I don't know why. I just decided not to."

But I know why. My grandmother had been indomitable in her struggle to support and raise her children. But she would come home from work and hit them.

"Don't hit, Momma, I'll be good!" they would chorus.

"Where else can I take out my anger?" my grandmother would ask them rhetorically. "I can't do it at work." Her children were expected to accept this reasonable attitude and the hitting that went with it. Apparently, they did. But while Mother never mentioned any physical pain she suffered from her mother's punishments, she never spanked me. And that saved her from me at the crucial moment. That one boundary, my physical self, that she'd always respected, had remained in place at the climactic moment when we both needed it most.

But next time we might not be so lucky. A week later I voluntarily signed in to a halfway mental hospital Mother located. I'd scared both of us. I had to get out of her house. This was the only place to go.

I lasted there six weeks.

The lithium they gave me pasted numbness over my brain. But beneath the anesthetizing sensation, I could still hear in my head my frantic screams of anger and pain, and I wanted access to them. I wanted to feel what I felt. After my first day in the mental hospital, I refused more drugs. I wasn't into vitamins yet but felt obligated to take some kind of pill so I took a vitamin.

What got me kicked out was their instruction that I do jumping jacks with "the group" at seven in the morning. I was eighteen and certain aspects of my personality were written in stone. I wasn't a group kind of person, or a jumping jacks kind of person, and I was so-o-o-o-o not a seven-in-the-morning kind of person.

The rather senile psychiatrist, who saw me for fifteen minutes a week with constant interruptions from the nurses, told me, "You aren't conforming to our rules. You'll have to leave."

The place was getting depressing anyway. It was filled with depressed people, after all. So I left.

Out

Mother signed me up for government assistance and helped me find an apartment. Each time she drove me and more of my effects to it, she demanded, as she sometimes did in our brief, periodic phone conversations, and would continue to do for years, to know what she'd done wrong, even as she continued doing it. And just as I would continue to do, I fell for her reputed desire to know, promptly reminding her of her most common condemnation "There's something *radically wrong* with you!"

Her retort was emphatic. "I never said that."

"What? You just said it last week!"

"I certainly did not!"

"Okay, fine." I crossed my arms, the old anger immediately clenching my veins. I reminded her about the smile. "Other People are always more important than me. *Their* feelings, *their* needs. If I don't smile, I'm not good enough. I have to grovel to make them like me. 'Smile or People won't like you!'"

Her voice scraped the lower notes as if to indicate the depth of her sincerity and my inaccuracy. *"Oh, you're crazy! I never said that."*

Crazy! I'd forgotten that one. The truth defined me as crazy! But my compulsive smile tormented me! Why couldn't she admit she'd put it there? Mother herself smiled all the time, among Other People.

But the more driven Mother became to absolve herself of blame for my anger, the more intent I grew to nail it on her. On our next trip to my new apartment, when she brought up my unfair anger toward her, I repeated those rashes of "You failed me/I failed you." "No matter who failed who," I tried to explain, "I was at the center of the whole failure, and I was a child."

"Oh, no, you only imagined me saying that." Then she bore down with true energy. "It's who failed *whom*, dear."

"Why should I tell you anything?" I exploded. "You don't care!"

"Oh, you don't mean that."

I could barely resist the impulse to whack my head against the car window a few times. Yet when Mother again demanded the reasons for my anger, I still cradled a last, irate yet tender morsel of hope. Was my mother going to listen to me *this time?* Because I was *not* going to do this again! Resurrecting for her the Jewish holiday when I was menstruating, I mimicked her accusation to the last nuance. "'Oh my God!' you said, '*Smile!* What's *wronggg* with you? You look like a gloomy, damp, dank, dark, UGLY ***THUNDERCLOUD!'"***

"Oh," and she waved a dismissive hand, "those were just words."

***

The first apartment I got was too dark; the next, a few months later, overrun with drug dealers; another exiled me to the sleazier east end of Hollywood Boulevard, and so on. But after two years and several moves, I discovered a place halfway between Hollywood and West Hollywood near an excellent intersection of bus routes. As I stepped into this bachelor, I saw it offered a bay window that looked out on a green, quiet street. Rent was seventy-five dollars a month and included maid service.

I swore I'd never move again. It was an oath that would wind itself in a terrible way into the core of our story, Mother's and mine, a quarter of a century later, when our relationship had become deeply loving, and our journey together was nearing its end, and I found myself unable to save her from the medical system from which, this time, she couldn't save herself.

INTERLUDE

1965 to 1975

A Meeting

After Mother's divorce from my father, she found romance with an attractive Mexican photographer. But he returned to Mexico and no one else she dated won her heart, although a few tried to bribe mine by bringing me boxes of candy. Her friends kept urging her to go to the Unitarian Church. "You might meet someone there," they coaxed.

Mitch's friends were simultaneously urging him to go to the Unitarian Church. "You might meet someone." His first wife had died many years before.

One morning after I'd returned from college and still lived with Mother, she at last succumbed to her friends' advice. On that same morning, Mitch also finally went to the church. This was the one and only time either of them went.

From the first moment they met, they knew they were right for each other. A year later they eloped to Las Vegas. Sometimes love happens, magically, and works. What happened to Mother and Mitch is, it seems to me, the radiant side of fate.

Freedom

While Mother commenced her new life, I launched into mine. The Smile continued to convulse my face but I began to care about things again. Seeking to reclaim my feelings and spontaneity, I went to therapy, read countless books on Jungian and archetypal psychology, and practiced Zen meditations. I called myself a Zen Jewdhist. I was always on the hunt for my "true self."

Fatigue also continued to hold me captive; among other things it terminated most of the part-time jobs I was able to procure. In one office still graphic in my mind, I Xeroxed a tower of papers, set it next to another tower of matching height, threw out the wrong tower (the one I'd just done) and, mind bleary with exhaustion, thought someone else had done it—and blamed her. At another job that still rattles in my memory, I chose to swap hanging tiredly over my desk for going into the bathroom, sitting on the toilet and now leaning tiredly over my lap. My boss fired me. "You go to the bathroom too much," he said.

To build my stamina, I commenced belly-dancing lessons. Five minutes into my first session, I folded into a fetal ball on the floor and lay there in exhaustion for the rest of the half-hour. But I kept at it and, a year later, I was working part-time at different clubs. I could dance for twenty minutes straight, although between sets I slumped, exhausted, in a chair, waiting for my next turn. Also, even as my body undulated and shimmied and shook, I lacked that last ounce of energy I needed to smile. Belly-dancers smile. My forehead crunched in concentration. Where was that Smile when I needed it? My audience complained. Then one day while I practiced at home, intense pain crackled through my back. A muscle spasm twisted me into a curlicue. I could hardly stand, let alone walk, for two weeks.

Frightened by my pain and the diagnosis of tight muscles, loose ligaments and a weak lower back, I lay off exercise for a year then tried to resuscitate my stamina again, unaware that my mother was my inspiration for my continuing efforts; she took exercise classes her entire adult life. This time I started running around the block, then blocks. But six or eight months after I began, my back went out again. This time recovery took a month. My next exercise effort a few months later was swimming. Building my stamina, I swam for a year, until the pool closed. I swam at the next pool for another year. Then I saw them pouring chlorine into the water while we swam in it (me, gasping open-mouthed while I dodged the heavy, muscular arms of guys doing the butterfly on either side of my narrow lane). The pool I found after that erected a final impasse: I had to take two buses to get there. I was so exhausted when I arrived that I couldn't swim.

***

For my final and longest job, I worked part-time as a concession stand salesperson at a small local theater. During a Monty Python film, there arrived a ghost from my past. A tall, very attractive Black woman came out for popcorn. I asked her, "How is the movie?" We discussed it. She was smart and very funny. She lived in the neighborhood and attended the theater frequently. We talked whenever she came to see a movie. Eventually Rita and I exchanged numbers. Twenty years later, as we talked on the phone sharing various life experiences, I related my college crush on the exceptional Tim, who'd had a crush on a beautiful Black woman.

"That was me!" Surprise beamed from her voice.

"Are you kidding?" I echoed her astonishment. We discussed the details until we conclusively confirmed that she, indeed, in her youth, had been the woman Tim loved.

Five years after I began the theater job, my boss retired. His son took over and cut corners. The hot dog machine needed to be fixed. I said, “These hot dogs are green. I can’t sell green hot dogs.” I didn’t sell them. He didn’t fix the machine. Two weeks later I was fired.

Acting vs. Writing

Along with fatigue, my compulsive eating persisted despite my escape from Mother. Within a month of moving into my first apartment, I returned to the LAAT. I tried out for the plays, but I'd ballooned into a blimp. Fifty pounds overweight, unable to get any roles, I took tickets at the productions. At home each night I wept, pleading to whatever deity might listen. *Please help me stop eating!!* I'd loved acting my whole life. *I don't want to give up acting! I'll give a role everything!* But after a couple of briny-eyed hours I'd go into the bathroom, blow my nose and catch sight of myself in the mirror. My chin still twitched from crying and a bit of drool edged my mouth, which grimaced at the reflection of my spent, runny-nosed, tear-stained, less-than-star-quality visage. Demoralized, I wondered if, should Don cast me in something, I could even pull it off with my abysmal energy level.

Moreover, my nocturnal bus rides from an LAAT class or field trip, back to my various consecutive apartments, bristled with danger. I often left a movie we'd seen and our restaurant discussion afterwards at midnight. I waited alone on the bus bench, cold and lonely, while men with hooded leers pulled over to offer me a ride. I jumped up and stood behind the bench until they drove off into the dark, empty street. I arrived home around two.

I started to write. I didn't have to be thin or go out at night to write. Two years after I returned to the LAAT, humiliated by my body and defeated by those midnight bus rides, I quit. Shortly afterwards, a block from my final apartment, I found the belly-dancing teacher. I danced half my big ass off before my back spasm caused me to give that up, but my hips and thighs still overflowed chairs and stools. And I still didn't know what caused my fatigue.

In my late twenties Mother found and paid for my visit to an endocrinologist who discovered I had a thyroid disease. The thyroid medication improved my energy a little. Then I went to a nutritionist. Again, Mother paid.

A homely woman with bowl-cut hair, the nutritionist recommended the six-hour glucose tolerance test. I fasted and consumed sugar once an hour. I nearly passed out during the fifth hour. "You have hypoglycemia," the nutritionist informed me afterwards, "and an addictive allergy to sugar. You have to stop eating sugar and white flour. It overstimulates your pancreas to produce insulin, you get a sugar high, then your blood sugar drops to below normal because your pancreas is exhausted. Then you crave more sugar. It's a cycle. You have to give up sugar."

I stared at her. *"Completely?"*

She nodded.

I continued to stare at her. I ruminated about jelly donuts, pumpkin cheesecake, carrot cake, rich frosting. I could eat frosting until I passed out. (In fact, after a friend's wedding I'd stood by the abandoned cake, forking and devouring endless helpings of frosting. When I got home, I lay on my back, motionless, and stared through my glazed eyes at the ceiling for three hours.) "Sugar is one of the great blessings of the known universe," I said.

She just kept nodding.

Despite my thyroid medication, I was still always tired. I conformed to her advice. Nearly thirty years old, I lost my remaining lard.

Being thin was a terrific boon. Guys stopped ignoring me. A few minor relationships even occurred (all so brief they might have been submitted to The Center For The Study of Short-Lived Phenomena). However, while my energy level did not decrease further, it still did not improve much.

Whatever endurance I could drum up, I used for my writing, which required every functioning electron. My mother had helped me energize those electrons. But at the same time the old lessons, which I couldn't seem to unlearn, continued to undermine me as I forged my separate path.

Writing

I'd embarked upon my first writing project while I was still with the LAAT. A *Star Trek* episode, I wrote and rewrote it, each rendering longer than the previous one. My teleplay became a two-part episode and then a three-part epic. I wrote for two years. Then the series went off the air.

One big reason I couldn't get it right was that my core "wrongness" continued collecting barnacles to weigh me down on my voyage through writing as through life. Acting had given me the opportunity to experience my emotions and express my individuality through interactions with other actors. But the solitary act of writing was flypaper to my dread of my "wrongness." Since any genuine or intense feeling or action might expose that wrongness, I hid them from my potential audience. I wrote every scene and sentence in the reverse order that high drama required. The least compelling dialogue or action came first, followed by the next least compelling, and so on. My story built interminably toward what was really exciting, by which time it would have been impossible for anyone reading my story or watching my movie to be excited.

Moreover, due to my fatigue, I did most of my writing lying on my back. Years later I would discover that my concentration improved and I lasted longer physically when outdoors. I could settle on my apartment house steps and focus on writing for three solid hours. There's something about sitting upright and breathing fresh, even smog-choked oxygen that stimulates an alertness lacking in the prone posture and a stuffy room. Unfortunately, that was still the posture and environment in which, at age twenty-two, having lost my chance at *Star Trek*, I commenced "A Futuristic Yes-Play of Noh Origin."

I have no idea what it was about. But in months I had over five hundred pages, another saga, which I submitted to a prestigious writing retreat in Peterborough, New Hampshire, called the MacDowell Colony. I wasn't hopeful. I sent them a folder amassed with story material that was too intellectual and so rough a draft that I couldn't imagine anyone actually reading it. *But they accepted me.* I felt as ecstatic as when I'd won the poetry contest a decade before.

I was twenty-two and on a literal journey, a real adventure! Three solid days and nights of travel on the Greyhound brought my cramped body to Peterborough where I slowly uncurled and rose. I was too late for dinner and slept through breakfast. My fatigue dictated a special living arrangement. I was the only writer who didn't have her own cabin in the woods, a fifteen-minute walk, where lunch was silently delivered upon the doorstep. Instead, I lived in the main building, got up at noon (I already had minor sleep problems), picked up my lunch from the hall where it was left, followed my usual writing program at that time—lying on my back. During dinner I met several people who'd been trying to get into the Colony *for years.* My pride leapt higher.

Once home from my two-week exploit, I gave up my Yes-Play. But what next? I still possessed an unassailable drive to write. But what? When *Star Trek* went off the air before I could finish my everlasting episode, I lost the love I felt for telling stories. Hence, the Yes-Play, after which I spent the next years completing several truly awful screenplays of immense chaos and lack of grounding in anything that emotionally rang true. (Although they can't all have been terrible. I recall one agent I'd managed to attract who told me, "I always read your work because it's original. But you need to learn to write more like everybody else." I wondered what he meant but didn't want to expose my ignorance by asking.)

I had to write. Yet no plot or character compelled me. Not until the night I dreamed about an attractive young man swimming in a gorgeously colored coral cave in an underwater Atlantis.

***

After that dream, each day upon waking I lay in bed playing with the image of a coral cavern and bioluminescent fish lighting it while the strikingly handsome, gilled young man swam around and—did what? Why was he there? Over the next weeks an idea for a science fiction adventure about Atlantis evolved. The hero and heroine used their magical and technological powers nonviolently against an evil wizardly antagonist.

A passion for the story seized me. I was finding my new creative center. But I needed information to ground the story in reality and make the techno-magic believable. I discovered a group that met once a month to discuss the fabulous lost continent. But their meetings occurred at night, ending at ten. I'd require two buses to get home and be lucky to get back to my apartment by midnight. Again.

I called Mother. She was the only person available for the excursion.

Mother Takes Me to Atlantis

Mother had helped me move, go to doctors and so on since I left home. But an undercurrent of tension and hostility still thrummed between us. When we spoke on the phone a couple of times a week, her bitterness at what had happened continued at unpredictable moments to surface in an angry, aggrieved accusation. This provoked my own resurgent fury and continually threatened the precarious truce we'd somehow established. Although we never regressed to the emotional dregs we experienced when I was eighteen, my mother could always trigger my old anger and I could hear her unrequited resentment of it.

On the other hand, when she erupted into admonishments about what Other People would think of me or she burst into her old refrain about what was "radically *wrong*" with me or she started telling me what I felt, thought or needed, along with all those "You have to do this's" and "You have to do that's;" or she queried yet again why I'd been so angry at her; or her tone simply became adamant and commanding, summoning my childhood impotence and teen fury—I could, unlike during those earlier years, hang up.

Also, I wasn't financially under her thumb. She couldn't control me. She could only want to. She could only try.

As to getting together, after a few years on my own, I began visiting Mother and Mitch for dinner every couple of weeks, motivated more by a feeling of family obligation than affection. Yet a kind of companionship grew between us three as we watched favorite television shows together and talked about the news. And I could always not-visit for several weeks if I chose. Now here was Atlantis, a thread that potentially connected us to the better part of our past and ourselves. In fact it would weave into our future friendship.

***

Mother's leitmotif in life was "I love to learn." Among her numerous interests, lost continents intrigued her. Vanished civilizations, once-great cities, ancient ruins buried in the jungle, desert or sea, and the people who'd lived in them all captivated her imagination. Indeed, it was Mother's joy in these subjects that had originally enticed my own. I loved hearing about historical and mythical worlds, wondering about Camelot and embracing its utopian theme (the round table where all are equal; the end to war and to "might makes right"). When I was a child, Mother told me about the Arab city built into a red mountain. With her usual dramatic flair, she quoted a poet's vision of Petra: "the rose red city, half as old as time." How could I not be enchanted? And now I imagined my own version of Atlantis.

Atlantis beckoned to us both. Had it ever existed? If so, where, when, what was it really like, and what destroyed it? Mother picked me up and off we decamped to the meetings. Rapturous, we listened to guest speakers discuss every topic related to the drowned world. These included archeological finds in the Caribbean and off the Greek isle of Thera; ancient languages of the Middle East; the energy contained in ley lines; and the catastrophist, Velakovsky. He'd written that the Greek myth of Athena jumping from the head of Zeus actually represented an astronomical event, a piece of the planet Jupiter breaking loose millennia ago.

On the way home after each meeting, Mother and I jubilantly recapitulated for each other the new facts introduced to us. "Did you know that?"

"No, I didn't, did you?"

"Isn't it fascinating!"

It took me two years to complete my lengthy Atlantis screenplay. While I tried to sell it, sending out query letters, I began to write it as a novel. When that hit one thousand pages and mounting, I gave up. I got one actor to read the script but it was badly written. I knew it because other writers moved me in a way that my own work still did not.

I dreamed of making a living writing. My revivified love of story-telling continued. But I lacked the skills, and my fatigue precluded the hours of practice required for me to teach myself. Only recently have I been able to look back and see my wrong turns. One day after a few decades of friendship with Rita, we became close enough, or perhaps wise enough, to sit over a spicy Thai lunch and share those mistakes of our youth we both finally recognized. I told her, "I think I could have overcome every health obstacle and been successful in my writing if I'd known my craft."

"Did you take any classes?" she asked.

"A few. Over the years—two from well-known writers. But they were pretty inadequate classes, and I just didn't realize that excellent teachers existed or how much I needed one. So I never tried to find one. I thought I could do it on my own. The arrogance of youth. I just stumbled forward."

Rita confided that she, too, had failed to pursue important opportunities to learn and develop certain aspects of her song-writing craft for similar reasons. "I needed a mentor," she remarked, with clarity.

"Yeah. Thus do we all."

***

Mother's and my Atlantean interlude lasted a year, until the meetings stopped. That flammable undercurrent between us again came to predominate, though less than before. Then in 1975, when I was thirty and Mother, sixty (looking as if in her late forties), she told me she had cancer.

It did not occur to me initially that she might be facing death. Her diagnosis simply seemed another fact of life. Something you dealt with. But that sensation lasted only until I saw her in the hospital after her exploratory surgery.

Or did I really know the truth from the time she told me? My father had died ten years before, of cancer. I knew what cancer was. I knew very well what it did.

Favorite Parent

Acting, writing, pursuing health and my "true self": these were the trails that opened before me when, disgorged from the mental hospital, I was eighteen. The last simultaneous trail was my relationship with my father. When he first returned from Mexico, I was twelve. He lived in Los Angeles for about a year then went to Phoenix for a few years, trying to develop Olympics fencing students. Then he moved back to Los Angeles for the same purpose. His relationship with Mother and Mitch was friendly, but I don't recall seeing much of him until I lived on my own.

He would pick me up once a week and take me out for coffee. We talked about world events, movies and the theater. We shared the same passionate desire to become actors, he, regardless of the years during which it had never happened, and me, regardless of my fat and fatigue. Neither of us mentioned our respective obstacles.

We also spent time with his friends from Mexico. They'd moved to Hollywood about the same time I did. By chance my second Hollywood apartment turned out to be only blocks from Bob and Gloria's house, where their daughter, Helen, my age, visited with her husband and small daughter. Another couple they all knew in Mexico (the man, Carlos Rivas, a stunningly handsome Mexican actor who played the love interest of the runaway slave in the movie version of "The King and I") frequently dropped by as well. My father was renting a room with an old friend in Los Feliz, a one-hour bus ride for me. So when he wasn't taking me out, we met at Gloria's and Bob's, sitting in their living room, drinking coffee, eating snacks, Helen playing on the couch with her toddler.

One afternoon Gloria delighted me. "Your father never gambled in Mexico, or here, since he's been back." It turned out the only time in his life my father gambled was when he was married to my mother. I felt even closer to him. Mother drove him crazy just as she did me.

Another time Gloria said, "Did your father tell you about the bees he kept in Mexico?"

"No." I leaned forward eagerly, looking from her to my father.

"I made a little extra money that way," he said.

Gloria added, "Until the bees attacked everyone in town for three days."

They all laughed.

"They wouldn't let me start the hives again," said Father.

I joined the laughter, joy rollicking through me. This was my father: creative, eccentric, daring; just as I'd imagined. This was how his carefree side expressed itself, the side my mother found so irresponsible.

On the other hand, I wasn't stupid. On another day Gloria told me, "Whenever Helen had a birthday, your father got very quiet and sentimental. He talked about you."

I found myself sipping my coffee, oddly unmoved. I thought, *Well, why didn't you write to me* ***then****? When you were so touched and sentimental?* Since that disclosure I have despised sentimentality.

I also recall how, one afternoon around four, I was walking to Gloria's and Bob's, hoping my father would be there. He often showed up at their house about that hour. But half a block from their house I saw his white car pull out from the curb and drive away, leaving me with a wrenching ache of loss in his wake. I had missed him *by a moment*. He was always going away—to Mexico, Phoenix and, now, just, away.

***

As hard as my father endeavored to develop Olympics students, he could never quite surmount the barriers, some totally unpredictable. One night at Gloria's, she began the story of why Father left Mexico. "Your father was married to one of the most beautiful women in Mexico." I remembered the photo and little note he'd posted to me. "But he didn't speak Spanish," Gloria elucidated, "and his wife didn't speak English. They were fighting all the time. She decided she wanted a divorce."

"I wouldn't give it to her," Father said. "I needed to stay married to her to keep teaching in Mexico."

"But she had a lot of connections." Gloria laughed. Bob laughed. Carlos and his wife were visiting; they laughed.

"One day," Father continued the story, "I was going home. One gendarme came at me from one direction. Another guy came at me on the other side. Each one took an arm. They walked me to their car, drove me to the airport, put me on a plane and told me never to come back."

"That," Gloria finished, "is what we call Jon Wolf's famous flight out of Mexico."

I laughed with everyone else, including my father. But he'd been training students in Mexico for ten years by that time. That was probably his last real chance for getting students to the Olympics—and achieving a life of solvency.

I recalled coming back to my apartment once, to which he had a key. He was sitting on the floor going through a jar of pennies he'd collected, looking for a valuable one. I thought in pity, horror and contempt, ***I'll*** *never sink to that!* Another time, paying for our lunch at the House of Pancakes (still blimplike, I had not yet discovered my sugar problem), Father flashed a huge roll of bills, making sure everyone saw that he had money. I have no idea where he got it, but I thought, *Put it away! No one cares that you never have money or that you have it today. No one here even knows you.*

He was also developing, or admitting to, a devastating fatigue, worse than mine. I sometimes came back to my apartment from shopping to find him crashed out on the bed, which I myself longed to inhabit.

Only one year after I'd escaped from Mother, my father left again for Phoenix. This time he wrote to me.

Every letter concluded with some variation of, "I don't know why I'm so tired. I can hardly write." He had been teaching in Phoenix a couple of years when he called to tell me, "I have prostate cancer. I have to go to the hospital for more tests."

We talked for a while. I burst out, "I love you." It was the first time I'd said it since I was a child. He answered, saying for the first time that I could remember, "I love you, too." Both our voices broke.

I went to Phoenix. His tests were over. He now lived in the hospital. I walked into a large communal room holding twenty or thirty patients, none of their beds separated by even a curtain. When I located my father, I stopped in shock. His covers were thrown off and his penis was bandaged. An i.v. protruded from his arm, attached to the fluid-filled sack on a pole standing next to him. I went to his bed, covered him and sat on the bed. We talked. "So what are you working on?" he asked. The kind of conversation we had during our LA coffees and lunches.

"I'm still working on my *Star Trek*."

"You're taking too long! What are you waiting for?" He was angry and impatient. "Finish it!" He'd been writing a fencing book for ten years. It was still unfinished.

"I'm trying!"

Abruptly, his anger dissolved. His expression softened, as if he were giving something up. As if he were giving up trying to succeed through me. That wasn't him. It wasn't my father's style. A moment passed. "I know." Exhausted, he turned his head and gazed far beyond the hospital room in which he lay. He closed his eyes. I could almost literally see his spirit drifting away from his body, toward wherever it was he'd been looking. Away from me. I watched him through the tears that fell autonomously, as if separate from me, like a faucet. Father was sailing away from the land of the living. I thought, *He's going away again. He'll never come back this time.*

In the bathroom mirror I observed my tears falling and falling. I thought dully, *I need to go back out and meet*

Robert and Mimi. Father's brother and sister-in-law, with whom I was staying, had dropped me off to give me private time with my father and were waiting in their car. *I have to stop crying.* I stopped. Just like when I was twelve and had embarrassed my father, I stopped. But this time the tears only went into hiding.

I showed no respect for my instinct. I left Phoenix early that night on the Greyhound Bus. Yet I knew he was dying. I'd seen it. I leaned my forehead against the cool bus window and cried into the night beyond. I wept for the entire six hours of travel back to Los Angeles.

Robert called me two weeks later. "I'm sorry… He's passed."

I called Gloria and Bob. Gloria answered.

"My father died."

"We'll come get you."

That was a decade ago. For all that time my father, dead and alive, had been my favorite parent. But now my mother had cancer. No tears yet welled in my eyes. But my familiar distance from Mother began to shrink. At the hospital following her exploratory surgery, I stared at her. Her skin was toneless, her color matching the white-gray that had only just appeared at her temples and forehead in her fine brown hair. She turned slowly to look at me, an aura of weakness enveloping her. Her eyes held a distant gaze, reminiscent of Father's. But I did not realize this although I felt myself afloat on a sea of twilight, sadness creeping up from below.

Book Two

Reconciliation

1975 to 1984

Diagnosis

"How did you happen to go to the doctor in the first place?" I asked my mother a couple of years ago. There were gaps in my knowledge about this period of her life and a much-belated curiosity had begun to bubble up.

"Pain!" she replied. "I had a terrible pain in my side. At night I couldn't sleep it got so bad. I *had* to go." Mother was famous among friends and family for her procrastinations. ("I never would have gotten around to having you if your father hadn't pushed me," she confided in the last few years when she was sharing so much with me. "I was already thirty-one when I became a mother.") Procrastination was one of her traits that would never change. But right from the start of her cancer, another part of her personality, latent until then, began to emerge.

A few months after Mother's diagnosis and exploratory surgery, she was home and I was again visiting her and Mitch for dinner, now every week. Mitch would drive me back to my apartment afterwards. One night on the way home, Mitch told me about Mother's first, decisive meeting with her doctor.

"Your mother took all their tests and examinations."

Even more than usual, the words "your mother," like the words, "my wife," brought out a cherishing tone in his voice. "When the doctor got the results, we went to see him." I pictured Mother and Mitch sitting together in the doctor's office on their side of his desk, Mitch putting his hand over Mother's. "The doctor said, 'You have cancer, Hortense. It's a type called non-Hodgkin's lymphoma.'"

More than once I'd heard Mitch exclaim, "Oh, you can't trust women." "Women lie," he would say. "Oh, women!" he scoffed. More than distrust, I sensed he didn't like women as a whole. On the other hand, he genuinely enjoyed all my mother's female friends and, to whatever degree he held a negative view of women, it did not include my mother. "Oh," he would say, "your mother is different." *Your mother.*

Mitch told everyone he met about her. From clients (he painted houses) to anyone with whom he might strike up a conversation, be it in a store, at the swap meets he frequented, or with his friend, Walter, the mechanic, at Walter's shop. Mitch told people, "If I'd met my current wife in my youth, my whole life would have been different."

In the car that night Mitch recounted to me, "After the doctor told us, your mother looked down for a long time. Then she lifted her head. She said, 'Then I'll just have to fight it, won't I?' My skin shivered," Mitch said. "I'll never forget it. I never saw such courage."

My mother was the love of his life as he was hers. But when he witnessed her courage, I saw, his respect for her rose to a new awe. It emanated from his tenor voice, shaped his square face beneath the gray crew cut and dominated his entire being: my mother's courage inspired in him a deeper love yet.

For myself, I listened with fascination to his continuing narration. "The doctors cut your mother open. Tumors covered every organ in her body. They closed her back up. They didn't try to take out one of them."

Considering the aggressiveness of the cancer, the extent to which it had already spread, and my mother's age, they thought, what would have been the point? For the same reason, they offered her no chemotherapy or radiation. The lymphoma was Stage IV, the end stage, the worst it could be. Between themselves, we later learned, her doctors gave her a few days to live.

However, they were working with a new, experimental drug. With little expectation they decided at the last moment to suggest it to her. It would be her only hope. She nodded, agreeing to try it.

"And lo and behold!" Mother told me years later. "That drug stopped the tumor growth and gave me a chance to investigate other things."

Other things.

Her response to the drug was so dramatic that her doctors released her from the hospital in a couple of weeks. She continued her chemo infusions as an outpatient, a status that enabled her to step through an alternate medical portal that had opened for her at the hospital itself.

Kindness of Strangers

"How did you think to start investigating holistic medicine?" I asked last year, in my tardy curiosity.

"Well," said Mother, looking back. "It was most amazing. One day the door to my hospital room opened. A young man came in holding a finger to his lips. He handed me a flier. It was about laetrile."

"No wonder he had a finger to his lips," I said. Extracted from apricot pits, laetrile is a controversial substance used in holistic cancer clinics in Mexico. A major American medical institution once tested it and proclaimed it worthless. Orthodox doctors excoriated it at the time, in the seventies, as fraudulent. Many still do. "Who was this guy?"

Mother considered. "Well, he wasn't a doctor."

"No," I mused. "He wouldn't have been a doctor. Was he wearing hospital whites or blues or whatever?"

"Yes. I think he was wearing some color."

"Maybe an orderly? Or a nurse? Anyway, what happened?"

"Well, I already knew something about holistic medicine. I took vitamins and minerals."

"And you saw chiropractors." Over the years Mother had seen a whole range of sometimes ingenious and sometimes just eccentric chiropractors. On her referral I saw a couple of them, briefly, as well. "Remember that guy, Mal-something? I cried out when he snapped my neck into place. His eyes got wide and he stuffed his fingertips into his mouth," and I demonstrated, "like a kid who got caught doing something wrong. He asked me if I was okay. I said yes and never went back."

"Oh, no, I didn't know about that!" She laughed.

"Fortunately, you sent me to others who did relieve my pain without crippling me."

"Glad to hear it." She resumed, "But this young man in the hospital was really a breakthrough. I would never have gone to Mexico and that was the start." As soon as she was released from the hospital, Mitch took her to one of the holistic cancer clinics in Tijuana. Her treatment there didn't help much but she obtained a quantity of information, which she shared with me when she got back.

"The doctors there all think all disease starts in the colon," she said.

Aiming to fix this problem, she returned home with an enema bag with a hose like an anaconda, meant to slither *waaaay* up there and clean her out. The anaconda also, she said, delivered powerful enzymes to be absorbed by her colon to digest the cancer cells. Additionally, she purchased numerous supplements, including magnesium orotate, which she ordered from Germany but which is no longer available in the United States; a form of Vitamin A that by-passed the liver and made it possible for her to take 300 international units a day; more enzymes and other nutrients, including—laetrile. "Laetrile is an anti-inflammatory," she told me, "and it does help shrink tumors."

The more I considered her mysterious and benevolent hospital visitor, the more I had to agree with her about him. "You know, you're right. That guy *was* amazing." A young man had brought Mother a flier about laetrile, an act for which he would have been fired if he'd been caught. He had taken a great risk to help a stranger who probably wouldn't listen to him anyway. Indeed, over time, Mother acquired tremendous amounts of knowledge about holistic medicine and cancer, which she tried to share with others, only to discover, "Most people just won't consider doing anything different from what their conventional doctors recommend." So this stranger could hardly have envisioned the outcome of his risk and generosity. Opening the door to my mother's hospital room, index finger to his lips, he opened a whole new world for her. She read his flier and it transformed her life.

"Did you ever get a chance to thank him?"

"No," she said in surprise. "I never saw him again."

"'Who *was* that masked man?'"

We'd watched *The Lone Ranger* together when I was a child. Now she laughed with me again before growing serious. "I wish I knew. I only saw him the one time. He really saved me."

But she underestimated herself.

She saved herself.

Universal Laws

Perhaps due to the health-related accoutrements she obtained in Mexico, Mother lost little hair and suffered none of the terrible nausea common to most chemotherapy. However, prior to starting it, at sixty, her complexion had been astonishingly unlined and unblemished. But the first time she dropped by my apartment in daylight, I opened the door at her knock and was taken aback at how the chemo had changed her. It was as if overnight lines had broken out all over her face like cracks in a windshield hit by a rock or, as I imagined, a bullet.

I found my emotions further jumbled as she entered my apartment. Who was this strange creature? Just as when we talked on the phone, she shared her latest facts as well as the protocol she was working out for herself based upon them. "Cancer is systemic. It doesn't matter what kind you have."

"What do you mean?" I asked with interest and admiration. But I was at the same time angry that her precarious hold on life reawakened my love and made me exceptionally vulnerable to her attacks, and on edge awaiting them.

But she didn't attack.

"Cancer can localize as a particular tumor or system or what-have-you, like my lymphatic system." she quoted the experts she'd met in Mexico and others she'd begun to read upon her return. "But no magic bullet will cure it. You don't just zap this system or that lump."

"Then what do you do?" I puzzled.

By this time in my life I'd acquired a real respect for nonconformity; and as Mother countered the position of the entirety of conventional medicine, I realized that the very unconventionality of her chosen treatment provoked in me a wholly unanticipated sympathetic chord. There rose within me a familiar cheer, the same joyful relief I felt watching *Star Trek* when Captain Kirk tells Scotty to ignore some universal law, and Scotty ignores it, overturns it and saves "life as we know it."

Later I would understand that on a deeper psychological level, Scotty's success dramatized my own personal potential: I could trounce the ostensible "universal laws" of who *I* was and was always supposed to be. I could live my life as I knew it would have been and would be if I lived from my "true self."

But for now the victory was Mother's. She chose holistic medicine as the basis, although not the sole answer, to her survival—life as *she* knew it.

My mother, of all people, my mother, with her obsession about what Other People would think, became a role model of unconventionality in the most dramatic circumstance possible, literally as a matter of her life or death. Indeed, transforming herself became intrinsic to her treatment.

Moreover, as she went about it, she continued to share with me not only her discoveries in holistic medicine but the flowering of a new self; and our relationship, whose seeds of destruction had been planted in my childhood and sprouted their darkest blooms of deadly deterioration during my teens, also began to transform in its depths. Our relationship changed, in fact, despite the absurd ambivalence taking shape within me. At first it was I who resisted change even as, simultaneously, I embraced it.

Mind and Body

Mother's experimental drug was working so well that her doctors decided to proceed with radiation. Arriving at her house one afternoon to help with and eat dinner, I found her lying on her living room couch. She pulled up her housedress to show me her stomach with its round, tumor-enclosing bulge. A black circle was painted on it. "They put this black circle where they want to shoot X-rays. I don't know what the paint is," she said, "but it hurts my skin."

I sat on the other couch, at a right angle to hers. "When are you supposed to get shot?"

"Next week, if I'm better."

But every time she was supposed to go for radiation, her doctors determined that although she was well enough to continue with the drug, she wasn't up to radiation yet. Weeks passed during which I heard less and less about it until, finally, Mother exclaimed, "They've given up on it, thank God!"

Reporting what she was reading in her holistic medical books, a number of which she'd obtained from the Cancer Control Society, an organization that provides information on holistic cancer treatments, Mother said, "According to my guys, radiation is the worst part of conventional treatment. It's the one thing that's almost irreversible—the negative effects—no matter what you do afterwards."

With all her research, I didn't doubt her for a minute. I'd never quite realized her intelligence before. As she continued to share her broadening health education, my respect for her grew. But my other feelings remained less clear.

"Cancer's really a very complex disease." She elaborated her themes in another telephone conversation. "You have to address the whole person, mind and body," she finished, her tone reminding me of a small child earnestly mimicking overheard adult terms,

"Oh? Mind and body?" Despite my passion for nonconformity, when it came to physical survival, I wanted solid, left-brain reality, not airy-fairy "mind and body" instruction. *And this was cancer.*

Or perhaps my real objection to Mother's "mind and body" playbook was that it sounded *conventionally* New Agey, inciting my visceral aversion to the trendy, which I despise as much as sentimentality.

In any case while Mother was exhilarated, I questioned her extracurricular intentions. "How do you 'address your mind and body'?"

"Well," she replied, "you have to purify and detoxify your body, rebuild your immunity, and kill the cancer cells. You also have to re-examine your attitudes and relationships, reduce your stress and," she again earnestly cited her experts with childlike naiveté, "increase your joy."

I didn't want to discourage her from whatever she felt was right for her. But my skepticism expanded. *Not just airy-fairy but fuzzy-wuzzy.*

Or did my reservations here stem more from something entirely different? Maybe my negative assessment was just a way of maintaining the safe emotional distance to which I'd become accustomed. "Okay, that sounds theoretically sound. The physical part. But you're already pretty joyful, aren't you?"

I must have been more shocked by her cancer or her treatment of it than I was aware, to ask such a question.

***

How could I have forgotten her voluminous "have to's," all the things "you *have to* do" because life was so hard? How could her negative projections onto me have left my mind? Whatever she feared in herself, she saw in me—and, judging by my "radical wrongness"—what horrors she did fear! For that matter, how could I have forgotten for one moment the general nihilistic predilections she habitually launched from her downbeat side?

It was the "You can't," "I can't," "They won't," "It'll never" side of her, the "he/she/me/you/they can't/won't succeed," the "it'll never happen" side of her with its underlying, if usually, but not always, unspoken attitude, *Don't bother. What's the point?* No matter what suggestion I made to her ("Why don't you try such and such?" or "I'm going to see if…") and no matter what it was about, she automatically produced one of those negative pronouncements; and adult though I was, I still unfailingly internalized every one of them whether it referred to me or not, and all the more so when it did. ("Oh, they'll never" whatever it was, meant, "They'll never do what *you* want/suggest/hope/need/desire. So why try?")

But regardless of my initial resistance to her mind-body program, I soon realized that, to whatever degree a person's psychology is involved in their disease, the defeatism Mother sometimes expressed would certainly constitute a primary factor in hers.

Perhaps my temporary amnesia about her underlying pessimism occurred because Mother herself was unaware of it, and I, as usual, was internalizing her self-image, giving it precedence over my own perception of reality. Mother saw herself as a joyful person. The partial legitimacy of this perception further clouded my awareness. Sundry joys genuinely filled my mother's mind, and thus filled mine as well.

Joys

I recalled the joy Mother took in our very first television set when I was a child. She sat rapt through the series called "Omnibus," which I vaguely (but perhaps incorrectly) recall as a travel program. We similarly sat spellbound before The Hallmark Hall of Fame and Science Fiction Theater. And just as avidly she watched my children's shows with me. The puppets Cecil and Beanie brought her boisterous laughter. She often referred to her favorite character, Cecil, the Seasick Sea Serpent. Even now, in the midst of her cancer, she recalled and quoted one of her favorite episodes of "Rocky Jones, Space Ranger": "'And imagine!'" she paraphrased the hero at the end of the story. "'They did all this for something as insignificant as gold!'"

I hadn't remembered that. Her reminiscence thrilled me. Along with plays, movies and good television, Mother loved the invaluable ore of irony and suddenly I did, as well.

She'd also found illimitable pleasure in the concerts she attended, the vacations we took with Alta's family at the beach; the beach itself, where she body surfed wave after wave, the sun burning down; cooking and eating (she shoveled in jaw-expanding, morsel-spilling mouthfuls); reading the newspaper from cover to cover; and inhaling all manner of books from poetry (she kept a poetry book in her car) to an escapist historical novel series we read (the tales of *Angelique*, another of our shared experiences after I left home). She loved taking classes—exercise classes, Spanish classes and, of course, the Atlantis sessions we attended together.

But contemporary reality also captivated her. She found politics fascinating, and the global situation dramatic, scary, invigorating and riveting. Her self-education never stopped. And like my interest in ancient civilizations, mythical and real, it was Mother's passion and interest in world affairs that, well, inaugurated my own political awareness and minor activism (going on peace marches).

True, Mother and Mitch hadn't been going anywhere very much for the last few years before her cancer and Mother's own expeditions had only encompassed her exercise class. But she still loved reading books and newspapers, watching documentaries and music programs on PBS, listening to them on the radio, and taping every one of them, just as much as she'd enjoyed her previous physical excursions to cultural events.

But most of all she cherished Mitch and flourished in her marriage.

Mitch and Me

I wish I'd liked Mitch more. But it's hard to like someone who disdains you, and I felt the disrespect Mitch expressed for most women included me. Or perhaps it was personal. A slew of small incidents illuminated his disregard for me. One stands out with greater sharpness than the rest, and more coldly.

He knew how desperately I hoped my writing would get me somewhere in life, that I believed it was my only chance for self-support and self-respect, and that I worked at it as much as I possibly could, within the limitations imposed by my fatigue, which had never stopped. But one night, during what had become my every Friday or Saturday dinner with the two of them, I discovered the real attitude that lay in the reservoirs of Mitch's silence that charged the room whenever my writing came up.

In the kitchen Mother was cooking dinner. Mitch lounged on one living room couch while I lay on the other. (Mother and I had reverted to old patterns. She made dinner and I cleaned up.) The television blasted merrily before us, probably with *Carol Burnett,* a favorite with all of us. I said something to Mother about my latest writing project. I remember being excited. But a particularly potent silence radiated from Mitch's couch, cutting through the laughter on the TV show. I could feel him looking at me. His look was like a physical presence. Overcome by an unusually robust insecurity, I turned to him.

I needed just for once to gain some sort of support from him for my writing. While I felt confident in my talent, I wasn't getting anywhere with any of my stories and only two friends had read parts of my novels and screenplays. They believed in me although, correctly, neither thought I was publishable yet. The least I sought from Mitch was confirmation that he didn't totally dismiss my one hope for a normal working American life. But what I saw on his face was such a conspicuously bleak appraisal of me that I forgot about my fellowship to the MacDowell Colony. I could only think of one piece of evidence proving that my dream, however my health limited my hours of actual work, was grounded in reality. I affirmed with a kind of wild vigor, "I won first place in a poetry contest for my age when I was ten."

"Yes," Mitch responded, and before I could express my surprise that he knew about the contest, he added with the faint pity and contempt in his voice that summarized his overall assessment of my writing talent, goals, dreams and personal worth, "And it spoiled you."

I stared at him then recoiled into myself. He thought winning that contest had made me delusional. I dared to presume I might make a career of writing! That presumption was, in Mitch's eyes, contemptible. *I was spoiled,* like rotten cabbage. The rot smelled up the room.

I never again attempted to talk to Mitch about my writing although, stubbornly and rather stupidly, I talked to Mother about it when Mitch was around. I didn't want to be intimidated by his scorn. But all I did was subject myself to it and of course internalize it.

However, I *was* able to establish a superficial amiability with him, based in large measure on our camaraderie in the challenges Mother posed.

The Screen in the Soup

Mitch loved my mother for those qualities that my early experience with her had largely eclipsed but which I too was coming to appreciate and would also come to love: her intellect, humor, good-heartedness and naiveté as she burst with fervent eagernesses, explosive laughter, ardent exclamations and far-flung curiosities.

In addition, Mitch shared my mother's profound joy in classical music, especially opera, as well as the television variety shows they always watched together. Mitch was less enamored of news shows and politics than Mother, but his attitude provided a balance to hers. He'd painted houses all over the country and evinced a savvy working man's outlook that came through most clearly in the story he told us about a corrupt Southern sheriff running for office.

"He went on the radio and said, 'I have three big cars, a big house, a big swimming pool and a big bank account. You don't want to go through all that with someone else, now, do you?' He said it right out and they voted for him, the son of a bitch. What else were they going to do?" Mitch laughed. His cynicism was greater than Mother's, yet his sense of humor was open and without bitterness.

***

Mitch's appetite for food also matched Mother's. He chowed down her cooking just as I did, and just as she did. We all joked about her gustatory experiments and singular cooking quirks.

"You have to poke through the soup," Mitch warned me one night, "to make sure there's nothing in it you shouldn't be eating."

"Like what?" I wondered darkly.

As if on cue, his brow puckered in puzzlement followed by disbelief as he stared into his soup. He spooned an object out of the bowl. "Part of a screen?" It not only looked like part of the screen door to the deck but a highly corroded part.

I studied my soup, spooning through it cautiously. Then Mitch and I fastened our eyes on Mother.

She looked at the piece of screen in Mitch's spoon. She leaned toward it more closely and frowned, bewildered. Then, "Oh!" she said, horrified but laughing. "It must be the screen I use to make sprouts."

She showed us the glass jar into which she threw seeds then covered them with...a screen...before she moved the jar into a lightless place so the seeds could sprout. The screen, which she then showed us, to be used in her next sprouting event and health-conscious condiment, looked black and spotted with holes and in a state of general corrosion.

So that's how it was. Mother cooked the screen. Mitch found it and laughed. He loved the fanciful character of Mother's interests and eccentricities, and she provided them aplenty, thriving in the glow of his love for who she was.

Moreover, the things she did that made me literally crazy, Mitch weathered with aplomb. One night while I visited, Mitch asked her, "While you're there, would you bring me some cheese?" As usual, he lay on his favorite couch while I kicked back on the other and Mother puttered in the kitchen making dinner. Mother said, "Oh, you don't want any cheese."

My muscles contracting in tension, I involuntarily glanced over at her. A half-wall separates the kitchen from the living room. On the living room side of this semi-partition, cheap wood panels terminate at the top in a mantel on which sits a green lamp and some knickknacks. On the kitchen side the sink and counter stand. On that side Mother continued to putter, visibly moving to and fro in the kitchen.

Had she said that to me, had she uttered that oh-too-familiar declaration about what I "don't want," adult though I was, I would have responded with a sullen anger while at the same time doubting whether I really wanted the cheese. I turned to Mitch in fascination. What would *he* do?

On his couch Mitch rolled over onto his elbow, fixed Mother with a look of utter disdain and a hint of annoyance, and said, *"I said I'd like a piece of cheese."*

"Yes, sir!" She stopped, laughed and brought him the cheese.

The interaction was a double revelation to me. First, I witnessed Mitch not-internalize Mother's dismissive attitude. How I wished I could by now do the same. I also glimpsed their give and take in working out their marriage. Mitch would inadvertently confirm this observation another night as he drove me home after dinner. Arguing about some political point, Mitch informed me, in all seriousness, "What you say is opinion. What I say is fact."

My mouth dropped open.

I called Mother when I got home, and related the exchange. She laughed. "Oh, he does that with me, too." It rolled right off *her* back just like her telling him he didn't want cheese rolled off his. They had to be the perfect couple.

They even *looked* the part. If Mother reminded me of Katharine Hepburn, Mitch, with his crew cut, square face, and solid groundedness, resembled Spencer Tracy. Somewhere at the back of my mind Mother was *Bringing Up Baby* and Mitch remained amazed, befuddled and awed by her while keeping a protective eye open.

They were a pair even if he and I weren't.

Which was another reason that, initially, when Mother began the "mind" part of her cancer program, she confounded me by her stated need to find *more* joy in life. I asked, "Where are you not getting enough joy?"

"I'm not sure. But I guess I'll have to find out."

And with this statement I recovered from my amnesia. Along with the vast harvest of her pleasures that I recalled, there came back to me, with visceral force, the equally vast proliferation of "have to's." "You *have to* do this," "You *have to* do that, even if you *don't want to.*" "You have to *make yourself.*" I had to, she had to, everyone had to. Now she'd "have to" find more joy. Even if she didn't want to. She'd *have to make herself.*

But here was the strange thing. Her "have to" find more joy differed in quality from the soul-petrifying orders and edicts which, under ordinary circumstances, issued from her lips. The new tone was lighter and predicted the future. My mother possessed no awareness of her normally rigid imperatives, nor of her diverse negative projections on me, let alone of her defeatism, nihilism or hysterical attitudes. She therefore made no conscious effort to understand or remedy any of these parts of herself. And yet, eventually, dragging along over the decades, by some enigmatic alchemy, she made psychological transformations that matched those physical changes required for her healing process, which she had commenced immediately.

A Transformed Passion

The first thing Mother did upon returning from the Tijuana clinic was to create from her quest for survival a joyous exploration. She no longer possessed any literary aspirations. But with that same zest that once impelled her to "literally," as my father had told me, race home from the bus—and him—so she could write, she now threw herself into learning about cancer and holistic medicine.

She discovered the health conventions sponsored by the Cancer Control Society and the National Health Federation. She made annual pilgrimage to both, taping every lecture she attended. Between lectures she purchased books, collected fliers and pamphlets, and subscribed to periodicals, newsletters and journals, each of which further described the latest discoveries and innovations in holistic medicine—all those strange and consistently enthralling practices about which she told me after each convention.

Moreover, these conventions became her biggest social event. (Mitch had no interest in going to begin with, and his diabetes was making him increasingly tired.) She met and became friendly with vendors, speakers and fellow travelers on holistic paths to wellness. From every convention she returned home a fountain of jubilation. "I just love it," she would tell me for the next quarter century. "People come up to me and hug me. 'Hortense!' And I turn around, and there's somebody who remembers me from last year. They ask how I am. They all seem to remember me from year to year. We have the most fascinating discussions. It's the most wonderful experience, I just can't tell you!"

She continued her long freeway jaunts to the conferences until she was almost eighty-five, collecting information on cancer, diabetes and any disease affecting any friend or relative, and then informed and urged them to heed her discoveries whether they wanted the information or not. (My Aunt Grace recently unearthed a packet of Mother's letters. Grace has debilitating allergies and numerous other extreme medical conditions; Sid, Mother's brother, suffers pain from arthritis. In Mother's letters to him and Grace she goes on for pages about supplements about which she's already spoken to them on the phone, further spinning out her prescriptions, indicating when and how to take those supplements neither Sid nor Grace would ever try.)

But where to store this ever-burgeoning plethora of written materials which continually generated new files?

***

Throughout her adult life, Mother kept files. Already her three metal file cabinets bulged with articles, cartoons and funny headlines she'd clipped from every section of the newspaper. Now these health files materialized, fattening and multiplying over time until no room remained in her file cabinets; and there was no room for more file cabinets. Her health files, which nonetheless continued to proliferate, commenced to appear and pile up on unoccupied furniture surfaces, climbing upward like Jack's beanstalk until, reaching some indefinite upper limit, they commenced to germinate in plastic containers on Mother's small round kitchen table, encroaching ever farther upon her eating space. But what was one to do? What was more important, food, much as she loved to eat, or her files? She'd never been more in love with learning.

As much fulfillment as she gained from learning, she experienced even more, I think, from applying what she learned.

The Treatment

At her very first Cancer Convention she met an especially knowledgeable, and idiosyncratic, chiropractor. He led the pageant of those holistic practitioners who would become instrumental in saving her life.

Every time her chemotherapy sent her white cells tumbling so low she became ineligible for the next treatment, the chiropractor put her on a machine that was "contra-indicated for cancer." So he used the machine "for her back." (A chiropractor legally can't treat cancer anyway.) Interestingly, every time she underwent treatment with this machine "for my back"—she always placed it for me in quotes—she would then add in mock surprise, "Well, my white cells came back up. What do you know! I guess I can get another chemo infusion."

Equally essential to her recovery was, as she'd told me, detoxifying her body.

Stranger and stranger.

"I think these coffee enemas are saving my life," she said one day, a remark not calculated to enliven the odd dinner party or elicit serious investigation on the part of orthodox physicians. But I'd always been a little anxious about the unremitting fatigue that first appeared in my teens. I feared it might reveal a cellular weakness in my body that constituted a precursor to cancer. My genes compounded my unease. Mother had cancer. Before her, my father died of it. Father was only fifty-six when he died; and he'd suffered terrible fatigue in his last years. Had the source of his fatigue been the same as mine?

Of course, even in my late teens when I visited my father in Phoenix, I knew that his diet couldn't have helped his health. My hunt for breakfast at his apartment produced shudders. The refrigerator sent cold air over almost nothing while the cupboards swelled, shelf upon shelf, with canned foods.

But I wasn't eating all that well myself at that time or for a decade or so afterwards. So if I had bad genes, I hadn't done much to overcome the handicap.

My conventional doctor disregarded my apprehension about cancer as it related to my father. "You won't get prostate cancer." But Mother informed me, "Holistic physicians believe cancer is a systemic disease." So I could have inherited a cancer-prone system and fed it. If so, I now wondered, could Mother help me prevent the fruition of bad genes in a toxic system?

Part of my mind accepted whatever she did as perfectly normal, including coffee enemas. She was the one doing the research and she was the one with the cancer. And she was feeling better. However, another part of my mind caused me to raise my brows upon hearing her latest treatment; and, beneath those brows, with excessive exaggeration, I rolled my eyes. *Coffee enemas?* But we happened to be talking on the phone and, unaware of my ocular antics, she went blithely on to explain the reasoning: Imbibing coffee from the nether orifice enables the caffeine to blow open your bile duct, thus releasing toxic materials from your liver that have built up over a lifetime. "It gets rid of the chemo itself," she elucidated.

I began to yield to her logic. "And the dead cancer cells produced by the chemo?"

"That's right! That's just exactly right. I really think it works. I certainly feel better."

"I know you do." Still at the start of our changing relationship, I was startled by the degree of my relief in her rising energy.

"It's quite an adventure."

"So it seems," I agreed; although, I added to myself, in a tone of irony not without compassion, *Better yours than mine.*

Another bizarre component of the protocol she'd picked up in Mexico, and pursued religiously, I found even more challenging. When I asked what else she was doing, she told me matter-of-factly, "I buy liver, cut it into squares, freeze it and run it through my juicer."

"And—you *drink* it?"

"Of course." Humor in her voice.

"Of course." *Blechh!*

"They say," she explained with no prompting, "the liver has over five hundred functions and a lot of them are absolutely essential to the immune system."

"And you drink a cow's raw liver to...?"

"Support my own."

"Ah."

Her passion to learn and employ her new knowledge was equaled only by her burning desire to share her information as she acquired it; and I could not deny that, due to my disquiet about my own health, as well as my delight in her growing success, this sharing seeded one of the strongest bonds in our new relationship.

But Mitch was a mystery. On my next visit to them, I couldn't help but turn to Mother's rock-solid, salt-of-the-earth husband to see how *he* was taking all this. What did Mitch think about Mother's strange course of treatment? (And she'd once called *me* weird.)

Now it was Mitch's turn to surprise me.

Weird Miracle Patient

Mitch was a meat-and-potatoes man if ever there was one. He loved Mother's successful culinary experiments, but when one went awry (the screen in the soup being only one example), he'd say to her, "Why can't you just give me meat and potatoes?" For him it was not a cliché, it was a meal, if you added bread with an inch of butter, and a few bananas. One Friday night I asked Mitch, "What do you think of all these strange rituals Mother is performing?"

"Anything that helps your mother, I'm all for it."

"But you seem like such a, well, regular guy. And this is all so, I don't know, *strange and bizarre*."

"Your mother's an amazing woman. I wouldn't be able to do what she's doing."

"You mean fighting?"

"I mean everything."

I studied him. Abruptly, an aspect of my fantasy about the two of them evaporated: that he was the grounded conventional one contrasting with her high-flown singularities. I realized instead that he and Mother couldn't have been so close had they been the complete opposites that existed in my imagination. The truth shone in the simple expression in Mitch's blue eyes as he returned my gaze. Mother's looming death and the fight she put up inspired not only his deepest respect, but the very peculiarity of her weapons elicited Mitch's unconventional side just as it did mine. (For instance, Mitch was not opposed to conventional religion, but he despised pious hypocrisies and was unimpressed by trappings. He'd once told a priest he wasn't going to be "dunked in that filthy water. I'll come back after you clean it up." Mitch concluded his story, "He cleaned it up.")

I wondered whether Mother would have survived without his love, let alone his logistical help. It was Mitch who went out and procured for her the mountains of produce she needed to juice along with the liver.

***

Occasional doubt still bombarded me from that side of myself that had learned to collude with Other People. Most powerful of the Other People were, for me, as they used to be for Mother, authority figures. Especially representative among them were the Doctors of Conventional Medicine with their powerful slash-and-burn drugs to fight cancer. While one part of my psyche totally accepted juicing as a primary tool in Mother's fight, how, queried the Other People side of me, the Expert side, the Whole Medical Establishment side, could *juicing carrots* save her from cancer? "Mother, cancer is a BIG DEAL. How do you fight cancer with vegetable juice?"

"It's the environment."

"Huh?"

"The environment in the body," she expatiated.

"What is that and what does it have to do with juicing?"

"I'm getting to that." She went on with excitement and impatience. "Well, apparently, when Pasteur said"—*Pasteur?*—"that germs cause disease, there was this other guy, Bechamp. He said germs are always in your body."

I was used to Mother commencing her stories considerably earlier than required, although not usually a century earlier. "Okay." I let her continue.

"Bechamp said germs can only make you ill if the environment in your body is toxic. An unhealthy environment enables the germs to multiply and mutate. Pasteur said on his deathbed—at least this is what they say at the conventions and in the books—Pasteur whispered, 'Bechamp is right.'" Mother paused, confused by her inadvertent diversion into drama and history.

"And juicing fits in here how?"

"Oh, yes. Thank you! The fresh juice apparently does a number of things to improve the environment in your body so cancer can't grow."

"Such as?"

"Well," she enthused, "certain vegetables detoxify the liver. Others tonify the blood. Different ones support different organs and systems." As she went on so logically, my hope for her continued to rise. I was also mentally stashing away her mounting stockpile of data for my own potential future. My father had never accomplished his dream of sending his students to the Olympics. He never even completed his fencing book. Was my dream of being a writer to end the same way? Would I be sitting on someone's floor going through jars of pennies looking for one worth fourteen dollars, and then die of cancer? My mother was becoming living proof against such an outcome.

Her latest visit to the doctor validated the fact that her improvement went beyond the subjective. She didn't just feel better. Her orthodox cancer doctors were so elated by her recovery that they were calling her their "miracle patient." It dawned on me that she might really cure herself of terminal cancer.

It hadn't dawned on me till then, not fully, that she was *facing* terminal cancer. But now that that she was eluding its grasp, sharing with me her knowledge and health experiments and, in the process, helping forge our new relationship, the fact that she'd come so close to death stole forward in my consciousness.

So did further, harmonious notes in our rapport as she progressed toward health.

Dark, Leafy Greens

"The books and convention speakers emphasize the importance of juicing dark, leafy greens." Perplexed, Mother added to her instruction, "But I don't know what to do about fruit."

"What do you mean?"

"Well, it's most peculiar. Some doctors offer proof after proof that sugar feeds viruses, fungi, bacteria, cancer cells, et cetera and so on."

"I can believe that." The nutritionist who'd advised me about my own health problems said that along with exhausting my pancreas, sugar screws up your metabolites and heart, saps calcium from your bones, and so on. I'd certainly discovered the addictive quality of sugar first hand when I underwent the ravenous cravings, erratic impulses and depression that escorted my withdrawal from eating it. But fruit? "Even the sugar in fresh *fruit?"* Was Mother saying fruit was just as bad as processed sugar? I still ate fruit. I *liked* fruit. Fruit could shorten her life? Even as a hypoglycemic, I was allowed fruit.

"Even the sugar in fruit," she verified.

Even more than before, I hoped I never got cancer.

Mother inhaled audibly, as if for her too such self-denial required extra breath. "But," she mused, "they all disagree with each other. Other doctors and nutritionists talk about the wonderful nutrients in different fruits and how good they are for you. How do you like them apples?"

I laughed. "So to speak."

She laughed back. For the first time since her operation I heard a small return of the gusty blasts of "HAhahaha!" that I recalled from my childhood (on its good side). A particular evening from that earlier time came back to me.

Mother and I had sat with her friends on their balcony. She opened her mouth to produce just such an unrestrained bellow. But sucking in the gigantic preamble of necessary oxygen, she swallowed a bug, gasped, choked and, simultaneously, started so violently at the uninvited insect in her throat that the canvas chair on which she sat collapsed. Everyone rushed to help her. Rising, a little shaken, she was soon laughing again, indoors, where we all went.

During one Friday night dinner, I reminded Mother about that episode. Mitch laughed. It turned out he was hearing it for the first time. "Oh, I can beat that," he told us. "One day I was on my ladder. I was holding onto the ladder with one hand and a paintbrush with the other. I sneezed. Oh, it was a big sneeze! My dentures flew out of my mouth and my glasses slipped down to the tip of my nose." He touched his button nose tip. "I reached out, snatched my dentures out of the air, pushed back my glasses and I didn't lose my paint brush or fall off the ladder. Oh, you should have seen it!"

As Mother and I joined in Mitch's laughter, I decided how pleasant was our warm rapport compared to the enmity of previous years. Now, during our conversation about the juiced fruit, our affinity continued to strengthen.

"What will you do?" I asked, referring to the fruit.

"I just don't know. This is very confusing. 'Is a puzzlement,'" she quoted the king from *The King And I.*

"'Is,' indeed," I agreed, smiling. We each knew that we both knew the reference and realized that as well as humor, we enjoyed the same pop culture references.

Mother finally decided to let herself relish the tasty "sinful" sweetness of fresh fruit juice and balance it with lots of vegetable juice. "Especially dark, leafy greens," she underscored. Then she added enough more information about the health benefits of juicing to make me contemplate doing some juicing myself.

I didn't get past the contemplation stage, however. It sounded like way too much work. Two bowls of produce would give you just a glass or two of juice, depending on how much water content the particular produce yielded, and

Mother needed to drink several glasses a day. Flood your body with nutrients, that's the idea; and in fresh raw juice, as opposed to the produce you eat, every single vitamin and mineral is bio-available to your body. Fresh juice also contains crucial enzymes that die within the first half-hour. To make any difference in my health, even without cancer, I would need to juice at least two bowlfuls of veggies a day.

I said, "The fatigue it would help me overcome makes me too tired to do it."

Mother admitted, "I don't think I could do it, either, without Mitch." She cleansed and strengthened her body via the Sysiphisean task of stockpiling, washing, cutting and juicing produce, cleaning the juicer, and running out of and sending Mitch sprinting back to the store for more tons of fresh produce, especially vegetables, so that she could start again.

I found my awe of my mother's daily heroism matching Mitch's. Indeed, I was not only awed and moved but mesmerized.

Personal Power

How, all my life, could Mother have been so obsessed with my smallest mismeasure, so frantic and horror-struck at my slightest imperfection, and yet she faced cancer with this quiet dignity and towering courage? Beyond our relationship, I'd watched her throughout my life as she went places, got lost and threatened, on her dark side, in what I heard as a whine, "I'm going to turn around and *go home!*" She never did but getting lost induced in her an astronomical anxiety. But here she was facing cancer with, one could almost say, panache.

A term currently in use has negative connotations. "Self-medicate." The phrase usually refers to people who, say, have a brain chemistry imbalance and try to correct it by "self-medicating" with heroin or a gin and tonic. But holistic medicine puts a different spin on the concept. Here, you collect all possible information about your disease and the options available to treat or heal it. You discuss them with your doctor. Then you make your final choice. "You take responsibility for your own health," Mother explained. "You do what you feel you need to do."

Coming from my mother, this pronouncement flummoxed us both.

She'd told me how, when I was an infant, she had difficulty producing milk. Her pediatrician ordered, "Go to formulas," and she did so without question. He was The Doctor. He told her, "Don't pick her up whenever she cries. You'll spoil her. Just pick her up when she's hungry." Once more Mother obeyed. He was The Expert. When, years later, another kind of doctor wanted to cauterize Mother's nostril to stop a severe nosebleed, she offered up the offending cartilage without question. The doctor burned a hole in her nose through which, from a certain angle, one could see ever afterwards. Nor did this stop her from returning unquestioningly to the same doctor with the next nosebleed.

Then there was the time that I was twenty and our mutual rage had only just begun to subside. Mother agreed to go with me to the psychologist I was seeing, to try to work out our relationship. He asked her how she felt about such-and-such. She responded, as she did throughout that meeting to all similar questions, "I didn't come here to talk about my *feelings.* I want you to tell me *what to do!"*

How was it possible that, facing death from cancer, she employed holistic medicine without the orders, let alone permission, of her oncologist (cancer specialist)? Once as subservient to doctors as a supplicant before a god, without warning Mother was revolutionizing her total modus operandi. "Imagine *me* ignoring a *DOCTOR*!"

"I'm trying, I'm trying."

Subsequent studies conducted by conventional medical institutions have proven personal power to be a crucial component in recovery from any crippling or killing illness. But at the time I don't think this was widely known. Mother simply became medically autonomous. Conjuring psychological strength as if from thin air, in her modest style she took on the medical establishment, personified by her doctors, and she triumphed over their uniform will even as she overcame her impulse to obey them blindly; and all without missing a beat.

Meanwhile, we found we shared one last health connection. Our common shock and horrified laughter at the manacles on the minds of doctors fashioned one of the strongest bonds in our new alliance. We were equally, and increasingly, appalled.

Her Doctors

Mother's orthodox HMO doctors loved her warmth and bright spirit as much as did her friends, both her old friends and the new ones she made at the cancer conventions. Her medical file actually held comments like "good sense of humor" and "pleasant to be with." However, the people at her conventions applauded her discretionary efforts to save herself while her conventional doctors just laughed fondly.

Always amiable, she laughed with them as they dismissed her holistic practices and she continued augmenting them. Taking her doctors' affectionate patronization in good-natured stride, my mother proceeded with her nutritional self-help, chiropractic therapies and her chiropractor's exotic machines. (He had more than the one that continued to bring up her white count but was "contra-indicated" in cancer.) She also kept appointments with a holistic physician who gave her advice, more supplements and some shots that were probably illegal; he's one of the doctors who has served prison time for using holistic medicine to help US cancer patients. Of course, she neglected to mention any of these treatments to her conventional doctors. They'd have had a fit.

What they did notice, and protest, was her DMSO, a solvent she downed as her holistic practitioners recommended for its anti-cancer activity. Among its attributes, it gave her so formidably unpleasant an aroma (in the vein of rancid garlic) that the nurses treating her nearly passed out when she came for her chemo infusions. They begged her to stop using it. Ever considerate, smiling, Mother desisted on the days she went to the hospital.

As she went into remission, her oncologists graduated from glowing about their "miracle patient" to exulting in their "miracle drug." Then they realized no one else responded to it as my mother did. The miracle stopped with her. “Why,” I complained to Alan, one of her holistic doctors, “do they never pay attention to what else she’s doing so they can find out what makes that drug so successful for her?”

Alan shook his head. His tone held annoyance, anger and the resignation of being an ex-member of the orthodox system himself. “They’d do better to study one person like your mother thoroughly than a lot of people superficially.”

Five years after Mother entered remission, her pain came back in the lymph nodes in her groin. Cancer had returned and was eating up those nodes. Her lower legs swelled from lack of circulation. She resumed chemo.

Ever since the cancer, she’d been driving all the way to Santa Monica to attend a “wellness” group twice a week as well as her usual exercise class once weekly. Her wellness group focused on relaxation exercises, spiritual practices and emotional support. But at sixty-five she was finding it difficult and stressful to get anywhere on time; she was increasingly worried about Mitch’s diabetes; and Mother was the only member of the “wellness” group pursuing both a physical and psycho-spiritual program, and her comrades there were dying one by one.

Along with taking the chemo again, she reduced her Santa Monica “wellness” jaunts to twice monthly, recognizing her physical limits even in pursuit of health; eventually she stopped going altogether. She also enlarged her volume of supplements, herbal teas, and fresh juice, and developed lifelong cancer-preventing eating habits, initiating each meal with raw veggies and dinner with a massive mixed vegetable salad. She also maintained her high focus on joy.

For the rest of her life, her lower legs remained swollen and susceptible to infection from lack of circulation, a condition called lymphedema because it originated with the loss of part of her groin lymph glands due to her lymphoma. But all her tumors dissolved. Her HMO oncologist periodically checked her and confirmed that she remained cancer-free even as he remained uninterested in the nature of her recovery, despite his lack of success elsewhere.

One day Mother returned from a visit to her new oncologist.

"Somebody new?" I was surprised. "What happened to Stuart?"

"He quit! He's moving into another specialty. He told me too many of his patients died. He couldn't stand it anymore."

Nonetheless, neither Stuart nor any of Mother's other conventional doctors, all of whose concern was saving lives, ever considered attempting to discover why my mother experienced this remarkable remission, as opposed to their less fortunate patients. Instead they persisted in regarding her holistic activities as mere, if endearing, idiosyncrasies. Mother and I never ceased to express to each other our amazement at this lack of medical curiosity, which betrayed both science and patients.

Fortunately, not everyone was so peculiarly incurious as her doctors. Once in a while someone with cancer heard about Mother, wanted to learn, and called her.

"I would never tell anyone with cancer what to do," Mother asserted to me on occasion. "It was just luck that what I did worked for me." Yet she shared all she knew with whoever asked and continued for the rest of her life to collect new information in ever-expanding files for just that purpose. She also kept reading and filing information to satisfy her insatiable fascination with the latest research and innovations in healing just about everything. "I'm absolutely enthralled!" she repeated time and again while her files on treatments for the entire range of sundry diseases expanded. She even came up with a few answers for me, including a supplement that eliminated the bone spur growing at the bottom of my right heel. It had become so painful all through my foot and to the top of my ankle that I couldn't put my foot down. A particular brand of trace minerals completely and safely dissolved the spur.

But Mother's pivotal transformation, in herself and in our relationship, was psychological.

A Different Smile

My mother's anxiety that should either of us fail to smile, global catastrophe would result; her steadfast unconscious guilt in enjoying life too much, a secret guilt she projected onto me; her belief that she was unattractive and second best, an insecurity that, in frenzied overdrive, she also projected onto me in the form of my "wrongness": none of these parts of herself did she ever see, question or deliberately attempt to fix. Yet as years passed, fewer proclamations and accusations sprang from her mouth; and those aspects of herself that I believed she could *never* change, transformed most vividly.

I remember the day I was reading Tarzan and Mother had scrutinized me with mounting tension, asking whether there wasn't something else I should be doing. But a few years ago in an evening phone conversation, I told her about some relaxing, enjoyable activity in which I was engaged. I could hear a nebulous frown edge forward as she said, "Shouldn't you be doing something—something—?" she struggled.

"More stressful and unpleasant?" I finished for her, and laughed.

And she laughed, too. "Yes. More stressful and unpleasant." She was laughing at herself. "You shouldn't be enjoying yourself like that!"

We laughed together.

She had changed to her roots, apparently by default. Her personality had over time softened at the edges, and deep within her the rigidity unbent and she began to let go. Or perhaps, paradoxically, the self-assertion she exercised in the medical arena gave her the inner strength to allow her outer boundaries to become more flexible, and luminous.

In any case from my mother I learned, at least theoretically, the two-fold lesson, which today I attempt finally to integrate into my life. First, it *is* possible to transform the self-defeating elements at the very core of your personality. Second, even in the face of a fatal disease, you don't have to be perfect in that transformation in order to heal whatever needs healing.

Perhaps more than anything else, Mother's drive to smile, to control the world around her by smiling it into submission, the smile she drove into me like a wooden stake into a vampire's heart, altered over time. She stopped ordering me to smile, and her own smile became wholly genuine. Whether she was pushing a shopping cart down a supermarket aisle or sitting at her kitchen table or on her deck, reading, her lips were upturned in a perpetual expression of warmth, pleasure and wonderment at the joy of life. This is the smile that seems to emanate from her house as I gaze up at it from the yard that once was hers and now is mine, the yard in which I sit huddling against the damp and cold.

I continued to visit her and Mitch on Friday nights, she dropped by my apartment for little visits and we spoke on the phone a few times a week. Only on the rarest occasion did I hear in her tone or comment her old bitterness at my teen explosion of rage: She had loved me *so much*! She didn't deserve that! She'd been the perfect mother!

When I did hear that tone or implication, I felt my old anger flare up. When was she going to let it go? When was she going to forgive me?

And, when was I going to forgive her?

Eventually even those moments cease to occur. For years we believed that our relationship was healed. Then there transpired another catastrophic event, this time to me. And our new relationship faced its essential and greatest hurdles: our old relationship and our old selves.

Book Three

Shiva

1984 to 1997

Justin

I'd met Justin a couple of weeks before. When I came home from shopping, an attractive young man was standing in front of my apartment house, slouched against a car wearing slacks and a sweater. To my curious glance he responded, "I'm waiting for the apartment manager to let him know I'm not taking the apartment."

"Wow! That's so responsible and considerate," I could not help but blurt, thus setting off a half-hour conversation. I invited him inside. We talked for two more hours. He called me the next day. We talked on the phone, at malls, at his apartment and mine for hours. We did not stop talking for three weeks. It turned out he'd been standing in front of the wrong apartment. *We were meant to meet,* I thought.

My mother was thrilled for me. While she could imagine me being happy with my creative life, and wanted me to get well, she also wanted me to find a great relationship. When I told her about Justin, who was possibly The One, she'd said, "Oh, I hope so!"

By the time Justin and I made love, I felt I'd known him for years. I couldn't get pregnant; I'd had my tubes tied when I was thirty. When Justin told me he hadn't made love much in the last few years either, I trusted him. We didn't use protection. Sugar Plum Fairies still leapt from chamber to chamber in my heart.

On the evening I learned the truth, Justin arrived at my apartment looking tense. He said, "I have to tell you something." We sat on my bed. I couldn't imagine what was wrong. We were going to kick back, watch the sitcoms and of course make love again, for the fourth time. Instead, he told me about Philip, his best friend who had died six months earlier. "Philip was my lover. He died of AIDS."

My breath froze halfway up my chest. I stared at him.

"The doctors told me he died of an AIDS-related form of cancer," he went on, "but it wasn't AIDS."

"He what?"

"There were some strange things about his death." Justin was defensive. "The hospital wouldn't release his autopsy report. His parents sued the hospital. They only just got the report." He held up a letter. "It was AIDS."

The small room that constituted my apartment shrank away from me. *This can't be real.* "What strange things? And why didn't you tell me you're bisexual?"

"I'm not bisexual."

"You slept with another guy!"

"It was just him, my best friend."

"He was your *lover."*

"He was my best friend. I'm not homosexual!"

"We could have used a condom!"

Although news reporters only spoke of AIDS as a homosexual disease, and said that only gay men got AIDS, I'd thought, watching those reports, that that was ridiculous. A bisexual man who was infected could cross over into the heterosexual community. But I never once thought Justin might be a crossover.

When he left that night, I called Mother. She said, "Oh, I'm sure you'll be all right."

I wanted to believe her. But my stomach was churning.

Justin and I did not make love again. Next time we met I was afraid to kiss him. We both tried to keep the relationship going. But I was in a panic and he was in denial. "You create your own reality," he said, hiding behind New Age philosophy, which before had roused so many long interesting conversations between us. "You're afraid you'll get AIDS," he accused, commencing the deal-breaker.

"I'm afraid The Virus might be in my blood already."

"Only if you let it be there."

"'Let it'? AIDS exists!*"*

He retorted, *"Not in my reality!"*

Tests

But AIDS was in *my* reality, and the morning after Justin told me about the autopsy report, I hit dawn desperate for facts. That morning and for weeks thereafter, I phoned the CDC (Centers for Disease Control) in Atlanta. I thought knowledge was power. I was wrong. The information I gained was contradictory and confusing, and I found more than half the doctors I talked to at the CDC no less appalling, in their own way, than my mother's oncologists.

When I told her about these latest medical experts, she was as interested and shocked as she'd been at her experience with doctors during her cancer.

During possibly the most repugnant medical conversation, I was explaining to the CDC doctor I'd reached that day that Justin hadn't told me the truth. Suddenly reality dawned on me. "I suppose I should tell anyone else *I* might sleep with that *I* could be infected." The CDC doctor considered this for a moment then replied, "Well. You don't know. You don't have any symptoms. Why complicate your life?"

I pulled the receiver from my ear and gaped at it theatrically, but in real horror. My head spun. Why complicate my life? Gee, I don't know. What about not complicating *other people's* lives the way Justin had done mine? Doctors (at that time) believed the incubation period for AIDS (from the moment you are infected but show no symptoms until the symptoms appear) was six months to two years. I'd already told this doctor that my few encounters with Justin had occurred less than two weeks earlier. So he knew that if I were infected, I would not yet *have* symptoms. Was this the kind of advice doctors were giving to stop an epidemic? At the Centers for Disease *Control? Why complicate my LIFE?*

Mother was startled by this story. "I don't understand it, either."

"It's like there's some mental aberration in doctors. I wonder how deep..." in my fright, I stumbled over my words. "...it comes from..."

"From how deep it comes."

"From how deep it comes," I corrected myself, and added, "Or how far it goes."

She said, "I shudder to think."

***

Yet our rapport was not total. She continued to reassure me that I would be okay, but I wondered where her reassurance came from. (Or, from where it came.) She sometimes sounded, well, not exactly unconcerned, but somehow as if my situation were not serious.

Today my friend, Barbara, insists, "Oh, she was concerned. You don't understand because you're not a mother. She was desperately concerned *for her child.* She was *willing you* to be okay. She refused to let it be real *because* she was so concerned."

Probably true. But at the time my childhood revisited me. *"That never happened."* My teen years came back to me, when I was dependent and vulnerable. *"Oh, you just imagined it."* Coming on top of the CDC doctors' denial, Mother's blithe assessment sometimes made me feel out on the AIDS limb alone, and crazy.

However, the doctor who suggested I not complicate my life was correct that I didn't know if I was infected. Should I take the test? News reports challenged its accuracy. Suppose I took the test and it said I was infected. Could I believe it? Same question if the results were negative. And what would I do in either case?

I didn't want to know, let alone take the test and doubt the results. "What do you think I should do?" I asked Mother.

She considered, but what could she say? "I just don't know."

I also didn't know, if I were infected, how I could bear to live with my terror of the future and the illnesses themselves when they struck. But gradually the controversy surrounding the tests faded even as my anxiety so escalated that the stress of knowing nothing outweighed my concern about acquiring possibly wrong...or right...information. After six months insurmountable panic drove me to a major university medical center where I took the AIDS antibody test.

I called my mother when the result came back. I told her, heaving a gigantic sigh of relief, "It's negative."

"Oh," she said, sounding relieved herself, "I was sure it would be."

She'd been right not to be overly worried. I was free to continue with my life. For about two weeks. That's when Scott, a nurse from the medical center, called me to ask if I'd take a different test for a research program. Scott explained, "We've found that some people are antibody-negative like you. But if we run a three-month blood culture, the virus grows out in their blood. They're infected."

My stomach dropped twenty stories.

"Antibody-negative, culture-positive," Scott named the condition. "We're trying to find out how many people fit that definition."

Agreeing to join the research program, I bussed to the university medical center and gave them my blood. I returned every two weeks so they could monitor my other blood counts while we waited to see if the virus would "grow out." Scott said, "If you're infected, it will grow out within three months."

I marked the calendar. I could think of nothing else from the moment the culture commenced.

At first I couldn't even write. Then I started making notes on the story that might be developing out of my life, or death. I also talked about my fear with friends, acquaintances and strangers at the bus stop. I drove everyone crazy, except

Mother. She always listened patiently and reassured me that I would be all right. Sometimes her reassurance soothed me. But deep down, her mild tone, her very calmness, again evoked in me our past, and made me more frantic. I *wasn't* imagining my danger. It was real. I was justified in my alarm.

I felt more alone yet.

Barbara says, "She had a wonderful attitude about her cancer. She had the same attitude toward you, and she wanted you to have it."

And this was also true, at least in part. And there was something else I would learn many years later. Mother sometimes displayed what is called a "flat affect." She didn't always show the intense emotion she actually felt. I discovered this when she fell at age eighty and broke her back. Her doctor assured her she would recover. A broken back isn't that unusual in an elderly person with osteoporosis, which she then had. But the pain in her back was horrendous. While it healed, she would sit at her kitchen table with a cushion and vibrator against her back, reading until the pain subsided enough for her to go to bed. Yet when I, or anyone, spoke to her on the phone, you'd never know she was in agony. Her voice, with its "flat affect," held no hint of pain.

So while I waited for the results of my blood culture, Mother may have been profoundly worried about me, despite the absence of concern in her voice.

On the other hand, she rarely if ever called to find out how I was or how a particular blood test or other medical visit had gone. And she did express conspicuous worry when she spoke of Mitch, with his diabetes. "He's not looking good. I'm worried. The doctor can't get his potassium down."

I listened to her with mixed emotions, some rather shameful. Fatigue still prevented me from working, I'd never experienced real autonomy, never lived my own life, so far I'd failed as a writer, and I knew I was a drain on society. Did I now face imminent death? In my self-obsession I couldn't help noticing that my mother *could* give voice to her worry about Mitch. *Mitch* wasn't imagining anything.

I never considered that with Mitch, there was no question. Diabetes is a terrible disease. He did face death.

I told myself that if my mother wasn't concerned, maybe she was right. After all, Scott, the nurse, hadn't called me yet, and every day he didn't call, I was closer to being okay.

However, in case it all fell apart, I decided to develop some health resources for survival just as Mother had done before me. Twice a week I began seeing an acupuncturist whom I'd met through a friend; and once a week I saw a psychic healer. I told few people about the latter, a practitioner whom some individuals might construe as, well, airy-fairy.

Mother didn't.

I put aside my feeling that she wasn't taking me seriously. For one thing, would she listen so patiently if she weren't concerned? Moreover, our new sharing relationship was too important to give up, especially when I most needed her support.

I told her about the church where numerous psychic healers worked. She listened with interest as I described the quiet antechamber where I waited to be called, how its tranquil ambience was the direct opposite of the noisy chaos of medical waiting rooms. "I know people would think seeing a psychic healer is crazy," I admitted. "I lie on a table and Cher, the woman who sees me, runs her hands a few inches over my body for diagnosis. Then she holds different parts of my body and sends energy into them."

"Oh, I'm sure you're doing the right thing," Mother said. She saw nothing outrageous in my choice.

"I also do the energy meditations Cher taught me," I told her.

"Oh, I admire you! They used to have us lie down at the Wellness Group and tell us to close our eyes and picture a meadow. I could never picture anything."

I had my own variant of that inability. When Cher worked on me, I could feel the energy and I knew that moving, cultivating and balancing energy were all real. In fact, I was always surprised by the light, gentle nature of Cher's energy. When I was on my own, picturing/sensing energy moving through my body, my face scrunched up with effort, and the energy was thick and heavy on those occasions when I experienced it at all.

For the most part, however, when I meditated by myself, I just couldn't believe the energy I did feel was real. For, by definition, it *couldn't* be real because (as I believed) my "life script," dictated by my "innate wrongness," precluded me from accessing universal healing energy. Only other people could do it for me. Of course I simultaneously realized that if the whole energy thing *were* real, my doubt constituted an energy form, too—one that would block any flow of healing energy that I *was* able to generate. But I could never get past my seemingly inextinguishable belief in my inborn wrongness.

Facing death always puts you up against your greatest challenges. I was not only being forced to develop resources outside myself. I also had to face my deepest psychological weaknesses and confront them with fresh commitment. Sometimes this led to little upgrades in my consciousness.

One day through a schedule mix-up, a different person took care of me. Virginia was the most powerful healer I would ever see. Some years before I met her she'd had liver cancer. "I pictured little men going into my liver and sweeping all the cancer into buckets and taking them outside my body." Liver cancer is almost always fatal. Her experience had transformed and empowered her as a healer.

Rising from her treatment table, for the first time in my memory I didn't have to will myself upright. I left Virginia and the church and it didn't require all my will just to move. It didn't require any will. On the street heading toward the bus, *I had energy.* I realized, by contrast, that I usually felt as if I were dragging behind me a huge and incredibly heavy sack. It held my energy, which was dead. Dead weight, and I had to drag it everywhere, uphill. But now, suddenly, it was as if I were walking along in a bubble of energy and *it* was holding *me* up. I was inside it, and it filled, surrounded and supported me. I floated in it. *This must be what it's like to be a normal person,* I thought; and then came the stunning realization, *My fatigue is real. I'm not imagining it.* "I'm not a fraud after all," I told my mother that evening.

"I never thought you were," she said, surprised.

Indeed, she'd always tried to help me solve my health problems because she did believe they existed; and her exceptional character in this respect was one more point in our growing friendship at a crucial time in my life. For years my closest friend had told me, "The more you do, the more you *can* do." When I found that the more I did, the more tired I got and the less I could do, she responded, "You can overcome it if you want to."

I knew intellectually that it's almost impossible for human beings to imagine an experience that is strikingly different from their own. But only when I actually had energy did I truly see how incomprehensible my fatigue would appear to most people.

After Virginia's treatment I was euphoric. I stopped at a boutique and tried on clothes, something that otherwise would never have occurred to me. I was always way too tired to even think of trying on clothes. But with Virginia's treatment, it was as if someone had given me a ton of money, only this was energy on which I splurged.

Half-an-hour after my new energy emerged, it began to seep out my lower back as if through a drain. Within an hour I'd sunk back into my normal fatigue. But the experience inspired me to keep seeing Cher, meditating and doing acupuncture. I also returned to the Jungian psychologist I was seeing the year before; she gave me a self-hypnosis technique to enhance my energy meditations and gain confidence in them. I still didn't think it was in my "life script" to be able to save myself. But I did begin to feel myself actually moving energy and to trust that feeling. To trust that I was moving in the right direction. To trust myself. My "true self...."

If only I'd been able to ingrain this experience more deeply within me, it might have given me the strength I would need when, years later, I alone would determine the course of my mother's life.

Shatterer of Worlds

I was entering the final week of the three-month virus culture. I started to breathe again. I was safe. I had to be. Then, with just three days to go, Scott called.

When I heard the regret that tinged his "hello," my hand started shaking on the receiver. The caffeinated tea I'd been drinking all day sent a fever blazing into my forehead and cheeks.

Scott said, "It grew out in your blood. You're mildly infected."

His words twisted meaninglessly in my head. Finally, making sense of them, I forced a laugh. My old Good Little Girl Smile. "Is that like being 'mildly' pregnant?"

His laughter was a little more energetic than mine, or just louder, but just as false. This time the diagnosis was definite.

I hung up. I was sitting on my bed. Around me the whole universe seemed to tilt slowly onto its side. *I had it.* The walls around me, my furniture, television set, knickknacks, every physical thing in my apartment took on an alien underglow, a kind of eerie white light that resurrected for me an incident about which I'd read long ago. At the time I'd found it intellectually stimulating. Now it was personal. And it inspired pure terror.

The event was this:

When Robert J. Oppenheimer witnessed the first test of the atom bomb, of which he was declared the "father," an image came to him from ancient myth. Preceding the mushroom-shaped atomic explosion in the Southwest desert was a flash of blinding white light that went beyond all human experience. It occurred on the scale of gods. And Oppenheimer thought about the Hindu epic in which the god Shiva announces, "I am become Death, the Shatterer of Worlds."

I was alone in my apartment, with Shiva.

Who could have imagined that a major university medical center, and ultimately five cultures augmented by a bevy of appalling symptoms, could be even partly wrong?

***

I was thirty-five. Compared to where my health stands today, my symptoms then were nothing. But at the time they seemed overwhelming. So when I noticed—as no one else seemed to—that the news media was in error when it declared that half the people who became infected with HIV got AIDS (they *all* got AIDS), and that half of those with AIDS died (they *all* died then), I said to my mother, wracked by dread, "As unhealthy as I already am, I'm for sure one of the people who gets full-blown AIDS." I told her about Shiva.

She said, "My god, what a powerful image!"

"Thank you." Then, literary acknowledgement aside, I thought about the cancers, blindness, TB and assorted other opportunistic diseases and infections that precede an AIDS death. And I thought about death. I finished with a rising wave of terror, "It's been nine months since Justin. I could get full-blown AIDS *any time now*."

Mother said, "Oh, I'm sure you won't."

Experimental Treatment

Was she right? My infection was "mild." Maybe I could do something to get rid of it. When Mother called with exciting information a month after my diagnosis, my hope grew wings. She said, "I heard about an experimental treatment at my convention. It's called 'ozone therapy.' They say it's antiviral, anti-fungal and anti-bacterial. And it's completely non-toxic."

But I hesitated. "Will you pay for it?"

There was an abrupt pause.

I stiffened.

I was taking a few nutritional supplements about which I'd heard from my acupuncturist. Mother herself had suggested a couple more and paid for them all. But although the cost was relatively minimal, she always asked of each, "Is this really necessary?"

"Well, yes, if I have The Virus." But I pretended to myself that her resistance to paying wasn't there. I didn't want to believe it. Now I started to panic. An ozone treatment would cost more than a few supplements. "I could get AIDS. This could save me."

"Well," she said. Her tone carried resentment. "Then I guess I'll have to, won't I?"

I suppressed an angry "Yes" and fought back tears of betrayal. What had happened to the love she professed all the years I was growing up? What had happened to, "What's mine is yours and what's yours is mine" now that we were talking about what was hers? For that matter what had become of our better relationship? Without her help I would die. *You have to do this, you have to do that. Even if you don't want to.* Her instinctive reaction to saving me seemed to be that it would cost too much money.

True, she didn't accept my danger as real. She thought I'd be fine. So why put out a lot of money? But the ozone was her idea. She must to some degree believe that my life was at stake. So how did she *think* I would pay for it? But I saw that suddenly my need to survive drove her lifelong fear of poverty back to the surface and, legitimately, stronger than ever.

She'd inherited a large sum of money recently from a relative our family had stopped talking to, or about, but who'd died without leaving a will. The state got half of his holdings and his family got the rest, divided evenly. But Mother hated giving up any of her share. What if one day she needed it for her own survival? She was sixty-five with no future income.

But she was my mother. She felt obligated. And she *was* my mother. She really wanted to help. She did love me. I heard that, too, in her voice. That's why she told me about the ozone.

And how loving was *I,* taking my mother's money when she was so worried about it? What if one day she did need that money for her survival or just to maintain a decent quality of life? Did I still want those pancakes? Was this the same thing? I'd once imagined that death would take me outside my mother's orbit. But I was finding just the opposite was true. Yet if I didn't kill The Virus while it was "mild," it would kill me.

"I'll pay you back," I promised, still convinced that one day my writing would make money.

"Oh, you don't have to." She sounded depressed.

"I *will.*" But first I had to survive. "Thank you."

I grabbed at life. Three months after my diagnosis, I dry-docked my emotional qualms and flew to a Las Vegas clinic for the ozone therapy. Mother paid for my trip.

Our ignorance about this virus, as well as the ozone treatment, would prove devastating.

The Clinic

HIV, the pathogen that causes AIDS, belongs to a sub-group of viruses called retroviruses. What neither of us knew was that, like all retroviruses, HIV can't be cured. For a retrovirus insinuates its deadly gene sequence into your own genes. It becomes intrinsic to your very DNA, intimate as a demon lover. Treatment can minimize its effects but never eliminate its presence. And when the treatment stops working, the virus floods your blood once more, bringing back all the illnesses.

***

I stepped off the plane into a windy Las Vegas winter morning. Once I'd settled into my hotel, I called Mother.

"I hope it works," she said, her statement addressing both our needs.

"Me, too."

In fact my optimism was zinging. I had nine months of acupuncture and psychic energy work under my belt but had never noticed an improvement in my energy aside from the bubble of energy following my half-hour with Virginia. However, I'd only slept six hours the night before my flight and would normally have gone to bed upon my arrival and stayed there until my clinic appointment later. Exhaustion would have killed my curiosity, let alone any energy to act upon it. Yet, although tired, I prowled the hotel at which I would stay during my four-day treatment. Actually interested to discover my dingy hotel surroundings, I realized that I had more energy on a day-to-day level than at any other time in my adult life. (Later, when I returned to Los Angeles, I'd discover that the blood tests I took prior to my Vegas trip supported my positive, if subjective, experience. My white count would read 9000, the highest number my immune system had shown since I started testing at the beginning of my virus culture.)

At the Vegas clinic the nurse inserted a butterfly needle into my arm, through which she injected a clear liquefied form of ozone. As it cruised my veins for the next two hours, I thought, proudly, *I'm saving myself.* I was doing just what my mother had done.

When I finished, the nurse told me I looked a little yellow. By the time I got back to my hotel, sweat cascaded down my face and body though I felt frozen to my marrow. In my room I turned the heater on full blast. It must have hit at least ninety but I was still cold. By evening I was so weak I had to crawl to the bathroom when I needed to go. I couldn't stop shaking. I shook so violently I threw my neck and back out of place and could hardly breathe. My throat and armpit glands swelled painfully to twice their normal size. I called the doctor, who diagnosed that I was "detoxifying."

"Oh. Then this is good, isn't it?" I said happily, sweating away, gasping for breath, besieged by malarial shaking.

He concurred.

By the time I left Vegas—one day earlier than planned—I was so sick I could barely move. *I have to keep going,* I chanted to myself. *I have to get home and lie down in my own bed.* But I kept myself upright only by generating into existence second by second the last mote of forward momentum in the universe.

Friends picked me up at LAX.

Gone like a water mirage in the desert was my elevated energy level and immunity. The "non-toxic" treatment had blown out my immune system and triggered my retrovirus. Not like Mother, after all.

And the treatment never could have freed me from HIV in the first place.

Terror

My symptoms leveled me. My neck and underarm glands remained painfully swollen. Drenching night sweats soaked my nightgown and sheets five minutes after I lay down. I left daytime pools of perspiration wherever I sat. Bleeding sores exploded inside and around my mouth. My gums twisted and grew higher, making my teeth look crooked. A few of my fingernails separated from my fingertips. My eyes hurt and I squirmed from a horrific itch that attacked me from neck to toes. Anything that touched my skin, including clothing, sent me into a frenzy of scratching. As I tried to fall asleep at night, a vast slew of itch points struck at once. I convulsed so severely I verged on levitating from my bed. But I rarely slept. The itch aside, I couldn't fall asleep. In addition, a constant low-grade fever developed, I had raging diarrhea and my fatigue had mutated into a deathly weight that seemed to drag me with each step down into the earth toward my grave. By summer, my hair would be falling out, drifting over my bare arms like spider webs.

I needed help. I needed supplements and in huge quantity to get back even the health I had before I went to Vegas.

Once more I heard my mother's ambivalence, wanting to help yet resenting having to do so financially. Once more taking money from her gripped me with guilt. "Oh, my god," my mother said about every supplement for which I asked. "That so expensive!"

She still paid. I still let her, promising repayment from my writing.

After six weeks my symptoms eased enough to permit me to get out of bed. I started blood tests at my HMO. My numbers dropped month by month until my doctor diagnosed me with what was then called ARC, or AIDS-

Related Complex, or "pre-AIDS," because everyone who got ARC got AIDS, and died.

I also sought out help that would not cost Mother any money. I found chiropractors and an acupuncturist who charged their AIDS patients nothing.

"Oh, that's wonderful," Mother responded to the news, happy for me. I could also hear in her enthusiasm vast relief for herself. Then she addressed with some denigration other healers, those who demanded high payment. "Medical people are supposed to help people," she said indignantly.

Cher had not charged me, either; nor would Eetla, the psychic healer I began to see instead of Cher. For Eetla was the role model I desperately needed. My mother had used various modalities to survive terminal cancer. But Eetla had cured herself of an inoperable brain tumor by using only the energy techniques I was trying to learn.

I also went to Eetla because I needed help from someone who had cured herself of a fatal disease, and who was not my mother. I needed to feel the energy with which I worked freed from the echoes of anger and various emotional ambiguities that remained between us.

In fact, working with Eetla, I began to feel the energy that I "moved" on my own become stronger. My doubt lessened. My old life script persisted; I still didn't believe I could really save myself. But I kept working at it, getting closer.

Meanwhile, Mother now acknowledged my symptoms with a serious tone, although at the same time her reassurance continued with unequivocal, almost blithe, certainty. "I know you'll be fine."

But despite my energy work and psychological advances, on the other side of my incipient optimism, especially alone at night, I was a wreck.

Dread scuttled beneath my skin. I needed answers to questions I couldn't formulate. I clawed at walls that weren't there, and there was no floor beneath me. I was terrified of being crippled by a variety of AIDS-related diseases and ending up in the hospital, helpless and dying with protruding tubes and under the control of *doctors*. But would dying alone in my apartment, horribly, be better? I'd approached but never really found my "true self." I'd never lived from a self whose instincts, feelings and perceptions I valued and trusted. Consequently, when panic lashed out from my heart, tidal waves of such terror crashed over me that there was no me left.

One day on the bus such a panic attack seized me. My heart pounded wildly; my stomach went into the spin cycle. I had to know what had provoked this furious agitation. I looked all around me. I observed outside the bus I a heavy shadow lying over the streets. In the sky a huge dark—*thundercloud.* I could hear Mother's words. "You look like a gloomy, dark, dank, ugly..." My past still possessed me. *I deserved this virus.* I didn't blame Mother, or tried not to. My interior life was my responsibility. But this clinched it: I was failing. I could not crush my deepest belief that the HIV in my genes manifested in physical form, at the most intimate interstices of my physical being, the horrifying, terrifying, ugly, repulsive wrongness that I'd always experienced as "me," and that no therapy or meditation had ever expunged.

While I did all I could to survive, all I wanted was to flee my life, my potentially imminent demise, and myself.

Toward this end I watched television. In particular, at midnight on a local station, reruns of the original *Star Trek* played. I'd loved the show when it first aired. Since then, despite my failure to finish my multi-part episode, it had become my all-time favorite television program. But now I experienced the series on a whole new level. Instead of finding escape, my psychical travels with the heroic Enterprise crew illuminated my inmost truths and helped to change me, even as Mother was beginning her own next journey. Mitch's diabetes was getting worse. "Mitch is getting so weak. I'm scared to death." Mother would soon reach her own depths.

Return to Star Trek

The three lead actors welded my attention to the television screen. Their charisma re-awoke in me the magic of theater. Shatner, Nimoy and Kelley were each grounded in his distinct personality, which each transferred to the character he portrayed. That confident grounding generated a dynamic tension between the three that held me spellbound. Watching them, I felt scintillating within me the awareness that had first come alive in Don's class. *I too am unique; there's magic in that.*

But there was more than magic. In the face of my proximity to death, these powerful, highly individual actors and the equally centered and singular characters they portrayed counteracted my worst dread. Intensely observing each character's confidence in himself, I became aware by contrast of the feeling I'd been trying to escape: that I carried and deserved this virus precisely because I was me. But for those few moments during which I lived vicariously through those *Star Trek* heroes, I knew to my euphoric marrow what I'd always craved to know: *I am unique and to be unique is a good thing—not punishable by death.*

Then, unexpectedly, I discovered yet another tier of emotional liberation. Kirk directs his passion, resourcefulness and courage toward saving the lives of his friends, crew, charges and himself. McCoy also fights passionately for life, valuing the individual above all. At the same time Spock speaks for the lives and "the good of the many." Each of these positions mirrors and complements the others; and the personalities of the rest of the crew amplify the three main characters' passion for life

In this passion *Star Trek* revealed what remained as the central fact of my inner reality. I'd always felt that whatever I did or felt or what happened to me was unimportant as well as wrong. *I* was unimportant. I thought

I'd dealt with that belief, left it behind in therapy years ago. But my ARC diagnosis reawakened it – demoting me yet further: I found myself feeling that I had no right to fight for my life. My fight for survival was not only unimportant but a humiliating imposition on others.

But the *Star Trek* heroes constantly battle for life because life is good. Identifying with them I was stunned to find myself thinking, *What's happening to me is not nothing.* As these futuristic heroes wrestled for life separately and together, gratitude resonated throughout my body. I began repeating to myself, rediscovering this reality more intensely each time, *My life* ***does*** *have value.*

My new truths went still deeper. The *Star Trek* characters personified the very heart of the series whose raw idealism, bolstered by the cheesy special effects, revived my old, lost Gandhian ideals; my spiritual self; the self I valued.

Then, finally, in a series of episodes played closely together, Kirk, Spock and McCoy argued and fought to be the one who risked *his* life to save the others. If only while I watched them, my spiritual, physical and psychological selves joined together and freed me from my self-obsession. Immersed in these stories I was glad just to be alive and part of the whole human endeavor of creativity and love. In the face of being completely wiped out of existence, I experienced in totality, if only for those moments, the answer to my lifetime quest: *This is who I am.*

The proximity of death did take me outside my mother's orbit after all.

And while I made these nocturnal inner voyages, during the day I continued seeking sources of help that would cost my mother nothing. In this way I found new friends, one of whom took me on various adventures and even led indirectly to alleviating that financial pressure so dangerous to my mother's and my still evolving, better relationship.

Adventure

My phone calls in search of help brought me to Suzann Gage, founder and director of what was then called the Women's AIDS Project and is now Progressive Health Services. I told Suzann about my infection, symptoms and fears. She sympathized and came to visit me that night after her clinic closed. I told her I wanted to deal with my infection only with holistic medicine. I looked at her, sitting on my one chair, tall and thin with long straight brown hair. I expected her to tell me I was crazy. I knew from our earlier conversation that as a nurse practitioner, she counseled people who tested for AIDS at her clinic. If their results were positive, she presented to her clients every treatment available, orthodox or not. She whole-heartedly supported whatever choice they made. But to me she said, "If I were in your place I'd do the same thing."

It turned out that, for herself, she was totally committed to holistic medicine. "If I get in an accident and need to be put back together, okay. But otherwise..." She shrugged and offered to share with me everything she knew and would continue to learn about nutritional products and practices that might build my immune system.

Suzann became a source of profound support in my quest for survival; and Suzann, Mother and I became great friends. We lunched after every cancer convention. Suzann related information she gleaned from the talks that had occurred simultaneously with those Mother attended; Mother did the same; and I listened. Years after our first meeting, for the last Thanksgiving that occurred while Mother lived in her home, Suzann made an organic turkey dinner, collected me and off we went to Mother's. The three of us ate and talked up a storm. The next day I found some pins in my leftover turkey. I called Mother to warn her and Suzann to say, "You should call whoever you got the turkey from." I told her about the pins.

"Oh," she groaned, "I did that. I was improvising. I pinned the turkey together to keep the stuffing in. I guess I forgot to take out some of the pins."

The three of us regaled ourselves over the fact that Suzann the cook was just like my culinary mother.

But that would be decades later. Suzann's gifts commenced at the beginning of our relationship. She once surprised me with an invitation to a star-strewn fund-raiser for AIDS. One of the main speakers was—Burt Lancaster. As he made his way to the stage from the back of the auditorium, I approached him. Emblazoned in my imagination were his larger-than-life *Elmer Gantry* character and the colorful hero of *The Crimson Pirate*, which my uncle had written. Now in his eighties, about my height, Lancaster gave the appearance of fragility while a goodness emanated from him in gentle waves.

I introduced myself by name and then as Kibbee's niece. When he heard Uncle Kibbee's name, a sad, wistful smile appeared on his face. "My best friend in all the world," he said. Moved, I returned his smile. Then he continued forward to the podium.

Suzann was also responsible for my fifteen seconds of fame. At this time the media was just recognizing the existence of women with AIDS. From around the country they called Suzann's office, asking, with interesting phraseology, "Do you have any women AIDS victims we could use?"

We often did interviews together. Suzann took the role of Expert and I, the Victim. (The media people chose this arrangement, placing our chairs by category on stage.) Mostly with Suzann, I did about twenty-five interviews, including a Dan Rather special, a national radio program with Michael Jackson, and *The Today Show*. (One afternoon while I waited on the sidewalk for their camera crew to show up, an old friend happened by. We chatted. He asked what I was doing. I said, "Waiting for *The Today Show.*" He laughed. I asked why. He replied, "Aren't you joking?")

During my media moments, I experienced and expressed a wide-sweeping hope that holistic medicine could save those of us infected. But I was also thankful to be able to warn viewers and readers about the perils of unprotected sex: You didn't want to take the chance that, after all, nothing could save you.

In addition, however, even as I wanted to help other people, the media attention fanned my insecure ego. Outside my trance-like immersion in *Star Trek*, my life-and-death struggle still seemed as insignificant to me as it was to the world at large; and I still largely lived outside my "true self," frightened and alone. No one could get inside me and fix either my psyche or DNA. My mother's financial misgivings about helping me just made her human. But I still needed more validation. I needed the camera to validate the value of my struggle and of me. I often felt I existed more completely during my periodic media appearances than at any other time.

On *Oprah* this self-gratification reached its zenith.

A big heroine of mine, Oprah was becoming one of the most powerful women in the world. Suzann and I flew together to Chicago for our joint appearance on her show.

Upon our arrival, I called Mother from the hotel. "I'm here."

"Thank you for letting me know," she said warmly, otherwise placid about my biggest adventure, with an isn't-that-nice-dear manner. It was only later I learned she'd told some of her friends to watch me.

Oprah stashed Suzann and me at the Knickerbocker Hotel, sending a big black limo to pick us up for her show and take us back. Along with giving my ego a lift, the unparalleled reach of Oprah's show enabled me to follow, to a greater degree than anywhere else, Mother's example as someone who used her own health crisis to inform and try to help others.

But I have to admit I derived another benefit from my media exploits, with Oprah at their pinnacle: There's nothing like a little glitz and glamour to distract you from the daily grind of being scared to death as the phantasmagorical horrors of AIDS clatter toward you lickety-split.

***

However, when my fifteen seconds of fame went into FAST FADE, Mother forgot her earlier equanimity. "You were wonderful!" At the inevitable letdown following Oprah, Mother's words came at just the right moment; and I began to realize that while I wanted her to be as hysterical about my plight as I was, denial has its place. I'd been doing everything I could to fight for my sanity and life. I was developing insights and strengths. But there was one question that tossed me back into my limitations, and need.

No human being could answer this question. But I had to have an answer and turned to my mother. With my health history and current symptoms, beneath the confidence about surviving AIDS that I voiced on many interviews, deep down I expected that, despite my holistic program, the full-blown disease syndrome might well take my life before I experienced love, success or even solvency. I'd be just like my father, over whom I'd once felt so superior. My chance would be gone. My moment of life.

Every new symptom drove me to the phone, to the one person whose patience was saintly. "Mother, will this rash/cough/pain mean the end of my life?"

"Of course not, dear. I know you'll be fine."

"But what if I get AIDS?"

"You won't."

"Mother, am I going to die of AIDS?" *Cheep! Cheep! Cheep! Cheep! Feed me! Feed me!*

"No, dear, I'm sure you won't." Here, little chickie, open your mouth.

My mother's penchant for irrational denial, that had driven me crazy my whole life, now began to provide a balm. *I never said that. You imagined that. It never happened that way. It's just a dress rehearsal, dear, it's not life.* Okay.

It never happened and if it did, it's just a dress rehearsal. *It's not real.* Great! I'm up for that. Why the hell not?

I began calling Mother three or four times a week. I began to be delighted to believe her, rather than feeling offended and isolated. Indeed, I began to cover myself in her warm denials, to pull them up over my head; and when a fresh symptom or rush of fear obliterated them and I got cold, I'd call again. She never expressed one smidgeon of impatience with my calls or neediness. Whatever her shortfalls, she was there for me in a way no one else was able to be. Once I felt secure again, I could relax and find out how *she* was and what she was up to.

I know that despite her fights with herself, she would have come through for me financially had it been necessary. But, fortunately, a man of wealth saw one of my interviews and contacted me through Suzann. I shared with him every health resource I'd culled, which by then constituted a considerable list. He in turn offered to loan me the money I needed for my massive number of supplements. My wonderful benefactor died a year later (not of AIDS but side effects from the pharmaceuticals he was taking) before I could repay him. But by then my health had improved enough that I could cut back dramatically on my supplement intake, thus removing the most damaging area of stress between my mother and me.

But Mother had been right about Mitch. His doctor never got his potassium down. He was getting sicker. Then, hospitalized with heart pain, surrounded by five cardiologists, Mitch died of a massive coronary.

At his memorial Mother and I had an emotional squall that threw us back into our old, worst pattern. She appeared to confirm the feeling I'd had all along. She didn't care. And I finally had to make my decision.

Memorial

Mother was in deep grief. I felt only vague loss and, for her, sorrow. She held Mitch's memorial at the house of a friend of hers. Mother had always been at her worst with me in the presence of Other People, who elicited her hyper-vigilant awareness of all that was wrong with me and that might reflect poorly on her. Surrounded at the memorial by twenty or thirty Other People, Mother reverted to her old ways as if Mitch, and the woman my mother had become with him, and the two people she and I had become with each other, had never existed.

Various practitioners and supplements had stopped my diarrhea but on this day it came back and sent me flying to the bathroom. I'd been in there ten minutes when Mother began pounding on the door. "Other People have to use the bathroom!" she announced in a loud, embarrassed, angry voice. Humiliation broke out in me like hives. A minute later, my mother repeated her knocking and announcement with greater vigor.

Flushed with my own anger, this time I grew incensed. She didn't even ask if I was all right. I had this life-threatening virus, the ARC diagnosis and all these symptoms. Something could have happened to me but all she cared about was that I was embarrassing her with Other People.

When I emerged from the bathroom, Mother stood stiff, tall and tense, waiting for me with one Other Person, a woman I didn't know. The woman looked uncomfortable, not meeting my eyes. Half the people in the room were glancing in my direction with curiosity and embarrassment. I felt their glances as one mortifying wave across my flesh.

Mother glowered at me. I glared back, my face hot. At age thirty-six I skulked off, feeling as rebellious, sulky, helpless and furious as when I'd been a teen.

***

Days later I still couldn't bring myself to call her. But this return to our old hostility was a poison seeping through my body. Other than at the memorial, Mother was supporting me. My terror still underlay every moment and I still needed her emotional support. I needed her cooing every bit as much as she needed to be needed as my mother, and these mutual needs meshed neatly and added to all we'd learned to share, including a deep interest in each other's lives. She loved me with her imperfect love, as I did her. Did I really want to keep my old angry feelings for the rest of my possibly very short life?

I suppose in the end, at that time, all other considerations fell before, ironically, her gift at denial, which she bestowed whenever I needed it. But there was also this: Love felt better than hate. Warmth felt better than anger. My angry teenage self would always exist, just as would the corresponding part of her. But these selves did not have to dominate our relationship. I'd grown up more than that. Finally, I made the choice. I would have to remake and reinforce it periodically for the next few years. I also had to make sure to avoid all situations with Mother in which Other People who knew her might come within a light-year of us.

Meanwhile, the illnesses that swamped my body and the fear that ripped through me, sometimes accompanied by depression and despair, had inspired a new phase in my writing efforts; and Mother was there to be proud of my breakthrough.

They say you're supposed to write about what you know. Until my AIDS experience, what I knew was boring. I'd always preferred to invent fantastic stories and research or invent what I didn't know. But now I wrote out of the immediate emotional truth of what I was going through. The result was better than anything I'd ever done. I published for the first time, a cover story in the LAWEEKLY, an abridged version of the book I had commenced about my AIDS experience.

Eetla held a gathering at her house to discuss AIDS. On her front porch stood a high stack of LA WEEKLYs. *My* LA WEEKLYs. I picked one up. I held it in my hand. I watched other people pick up copies. I thought, *I finally did it.*

Later, when I heard on a radio interview about a terrific literary agency, I called the agency. The woman who answered the phone became interested in my story. She asked me to send what I'd written of my book. Within a month of receiving Part One of my unfinished manuscript, she was my agent and had lunched with a publisher who was eager to read my pages. If she liked them, she might buy my book.

That eagerness dissolved for a reason neither my agent nor I could have foreseen in a millennium. I discovered I'd been misdiagnosed.

Fairy Tales Can Come True

Two years after my first blood culture and four additional ones, Scott, the nurse at the medical center research office who first informed me of my infection and with whom I'd become friends, started injecting a mind-blower into our conversations: "If you even have it." I thought he was trying to give me false hope. It made me angry. It was one thing (in my emotional turmoil of a mind) for my mother to tell me I wouldn't die. It was another thing to say I *didn't have* The Virus. I had The Virus! After all the tests, *I had it.* I needed to deal with that reality so that the monster couldn't spring upon me from behind, when my guard was down. I couldn't bear to feel the joy of safety and life and then be slaughtered by disappointment and imminent, horrible death. I didn't want to have to start facing this nightmare all over again.

I didn't let myself listen to Scott. But he persisted. After about two weeks, I said, "What do you mean?"

"None of your blood cultures were specifically for HIV."

"What?"

He repeated it.

I stuttered. "Then what were those tests for?"

"They were testing you for reverse transcriptase." He sounded, in his subdued way, annoyed, or angry. He hadn't known, either. "That's an enzyme produced by all retroviruses. HIV is a retrovirus."

"I know."

"Well, they just assumed HIV was the only one. I guess. I don't know. Anyway, there's more than one retrovirus. I think you should go to a different medical center and get retested. For HIV this time."

A whirling dervish struck up in my gut, a dance comprised of genuine hope and all sorts of reasons for dismissing it. But I didn't. At the new medical center to which I went, the correct test came back. I could hardly believe the result. *I didn't have it. I didn't have HIV and, by extension, I couldn't have ARC and, by further extension, I wouldn't get AIDS.*

"I don't have it," I told Mother that night. "You're right. I won't die of AIDS."

"Oh, I'm so glad!"

After we hung up, I lay on my back in bed. Reprieved from my death sentence, I watched a dark cloud float up off my chest. Despite all the terror and despair dragging me down during the previous two years, this cloud consisted of all the additional terror and despair of which I'd been unaware, and had suppressed, and that I could finally let go.

***

My literary agent and I thought this turn of events would make my book all the more commercial. Who wouldn't want to read a happy ending? My friend Sharon, with whom I'd kept up all these years since high school, said, "It's like a fairy tale." But the publisher who'd shown interest in my book and those who followed preferred a victim, not a heroine.

That book would have been another fairy tale. A book! On the other hand, I didn't have HIV. I wouldn't get AIDS. And Mother and I had repaired the last vestiges of the breach between us. Our relationship could evolve for years now. And, actually, I did not desire to relive my "AIDS Years," as I thought of them, at least not as a strict chronology, which I'd have to do if I wrote about them. However, a related book idea began to emerge from those sanity-saving epiphanies that had come to me when I thought I faced death.

Resuming my midnight *Star Trek* vigils, I stared fixedly at the still-airing reruns. I took notes on the subterranean psychological truths and symbolism embedded in the series. All the different *Star Trek* episodes, scenes, characters, and aspects of the characters symbolically reflected my personal life during my AIDS years (the dramatic thread of my projected book) in particular and our shared human experiences in general. As before—but more intensely—the series mesmerized me. In short order, amassing untold mega-bites on my computer, I developed enough material for a large tome and, eventually, several tomes.

Year by year I wrote and rewrote, unable to give the project up but equally unable to coordinate all my material into a single completed first volume. After fifteen years, I finally had to admit I'd bitten off more than I could chew.

But just before I moved on to my next writing project, I did achieve one small literary reward from my effort. The C.G. Jung Institute of Los Angeles published a miniature version of what would have been my first book, a brief story of my AIDS "adventure" as it paralleled the voyages of the U.S.S. Enterprise.

***

The first time after my reprieve that I saw my mother, we gave each other a big hug, believing the story was finally over. I was going to live.

Jewelry

I was going to live! Or was I? What did I actually have, besides continuing panic attacks? I did harbor *some* retrovirus. Reverse transcriptase did circulate in my blood. There were four known retroviruses: HIV1, HIV2; and the other two both cause cancer.

Then consensus about the tests changed. The test most commonly referred to as the "gold star test" was once again the antibody test. I knew I needed to take one for each of the four retroviruses. Once again, I stalled until my anxiety at not knowing the truth outweighed the fear I'd feel if I discovered myself infected. When I finally acted, and all four tests came back negative, I was so relieved that I even convinced myself that whatever my retrovirus, it was harmless. Sick of facing death, I just wanted to enjoy my life; and I found unexpected joy which came as if from nowhere. Not far behind, Mother's latest change was similar to mine, a coincidence that, I am amazed to realize, we never noticed.

***

In the past my mother occasionally exhibited an unconventional stylistic flair. A picture of us on our one vacation in Mexico in the fifties shows her wearing a sexy, peasant-style blouse. That's also when she purchased her exotic Mexican silver jewelry, long before it became popular and achieved monetary value in the United States. And she gave me that satin Cossack shirt, which had been hers. But otherwise she bought the cheapest, most boring clothes for both of us, and they looked it. I disliked hers and mine. Probably for that reason, along with the Cossack shirt I loved, but which had garnered the patronizing attitudes of my college teacher, acquaintances and friends, after college I ignored clothing, and found jewelry especially uninteresting.

But liberated from my imminent death, I started getting up on weekends and haunting garage sales. A future streamed through my veins, and the form my rebirth took was as—a lust for jewelry.

This is how I met Susie (not Suzann), who has been helping me with the house. Stationed on her apartment steps several blocks from my apartment, she was a cute blonde. She was selling hats she'd made. I showed her what I had bought at other yard sales. After a few such Saturdays, Susie and I exchanged numbers and became friends.

A few Saturdays later I discovered only one block from my apartment another woman sitting outside the house she rented with her boyfriend, Al. They shared their abode with their mutt and a pit bull. Ensconced at a small table in her grassy yard, Margaret was selling the jewelry she made. "By hand!" I told Mother, agog.

"Is that so?" Mother was intrigued as I described my new acquaintance.

Margaret worked for a Chinese antiques importer. "I put aside a few little things," she informed me. "I keep some for myself and others to use in the jewelry I make to sell." She showed me her latest—gorgeous—"little things" from past centuries. Examining the jewelry she made from them, I fell in love with antique Chinese beads, particularly those made of turquoise or jade. When I was a child, Mother had frequently taken me to Olvera Street, a tourist attraction of Hispanic street vendors. My favorite people were those who sold little stones out of small baskets. Rocks and stones were magical. I especially treasured a ten-cent opal I'd singled out of the twenty-five cent basket. Margaret's beads brought back that childhood thrill.

I began to buy earrings from Margaret. For a while she seemed to become a friend. Mother met and liked her very much. But time divulged to us the truth. We came to know my neighbor as Margaret, the Thief and Liar. But Mother and I would agree on one thing. Mother said afterwards, "She certainly served a wonderful function in your life."

Before our friendship terminated, I sometimes accompanied Margaret into the workshop in her back yard. I watched her look around for misplaced beads and findings (ear wire, bead caps, spacers), and I thought in astonishment, *She's as absent-minded as me.* Then she'd take the beads we had agreed she would use for my earrings and rearrange them this way and that on her worktable. I felt a small, undefined excitement.

So she didn't automatically know the design she would use. She did not after all conjure those fantastic earrings out of the ethers. By experimenting in front of me, she demystified the sorcery of making jewelry, and in an unnoticed moment of inner fecundity a new image of myself took root—a possibility of myself. Somewhere at the back of my unconscious I conceived the idea that if one could experiment and be absent-minded, I too could make jewelry.

I always prepaid Margaret for my earrings. One day there was a pair for which I'd paid, that she wasn't making. She wouldn't return my money. So I asked for the beads. "What would you do with them?" She sneered. "You going to make the earrings?"

Margaret was angry because Mother had planned to pay Al to fix her roof. When Margaret confided to me that Al smoked pot, I told Mother, who decided to hire someone else.

"I told you that in confidence!" Margaret said.

"Well, what did you expect me to do? Just leave my mother in the dark when it affected her?"

Margaret had been storing in her basement two of the old metal fold-up tables Mitch had used when he took his own yard sale finds to resell at the monthly Rose Bowl flea market. Now Margaret, Al and I took them to there a few times. Margaret sold her jewelry and I resold a few things I'd picked up at yard sales. When I got too tired to accompany them, Margaret and Al went to the Rose Bowl without me, still using Mother's tables. Now I asked for them. Margaret refused to give them to either Mother or me. When another neighbor told me Margaret and Al were moving, I realized she was planning on keeping my beads, my money and Mother's tables.

Margaret denied it. "I don't know who told you we're moving. We're not moving. There are just some things in front of the tables. I can't get them out right now. And I'm waiting for some findings to come in the mail for your earrings before I can make them."

She'd once laughed privately that her little mutt "growls when Al comes near me in bed. My little dog is teaching—" and she named her pit bull, "to growl at Al, too. When I'm in bed." She'd laughed again.

Hmm, I'd thought.

I'd told my mother the story. Now she exclaimed, as we bemoaned the devious human pair and pictured the canine lessons completed, "Oh, wouldn't that be perfect justice! Maybe we'll read about them."

"Wouldn't that be nice?" I agreed, my Gandhian ideals left in the dust.

Mother and I continued to masticate the details, discussing that couple we'd never forget and, in the process, continuing to move farther yet into our new habit of friendship—of love.

The day Margaret and Al were loading their belongings into a U-Haul, I happened by. My mother's green metal tables were stacked outside. Al was not around, only Margaret. I said with an energetic smile, "Oh, you have my tables." I clutched the handles hard, one per hand, and paused with a bright smile while surreptitiously scanning her house through the open door and the open truck interior, where Margaret stood, for evidence of Al or the pit bull. Seeing nothing, I said, "Thanks." She nodded vaguely, with a hint of guilt—she knew my mother had really liked her—and of surrender before my cheerful, deliberate innocence. I carted the heavy tables off toward home before Al or the dogs appeared.

My hands were painful and swollen for the next few days. The pain reminded me of the extreme ache in my upper arms that developed when I'd gotten exhausted at the Rose Bowl. I suspected these symptoms belonged to my retrovirus but wasn't worried. So I had a little extra pain now and then. It went away. "I got your tables back," I told Mother that night. When I explained how, she clapped and laughed.

A few weeks later, as I meandered through a local swap meet (if I'd loved them when Mitch was alive, we might have had a whole different relationship), I spied a man of middle age selling bags of glass beads. I bought one. At home on the floor (there was no room for a table) I experimented as I'd seen Margaret do, moving the beads around into different combinations. When I had a few designs I liked, I took them to a bead store. The proprietress pointed out the tools I would need to make earrings and showed me how to use them. Before I knew it, I'd bought tons more hideous glass and stone beads at the flea market.

Since jewelry had never interested me, I knew nothing about it. It took me ages to develop any knowledge or taste. Then at last came a little skill. Finally, years after my reprieve from HIV and AIDS, my celebration of life had taken the form of making beautiful jewelry. In little fairy tales and major epics of pearls and tourmaline, sunstone and moonstone, turquoise and coral, aquamarine and garnet mixed with beautiful vintage glass, I put together the necklaces and earrings in which my mother and I delighted. Whenever we got together, she literally applauded my latest design, even as she underwent her own chrysalis.

She'd survived her cancer, my AIDS years and Mitch's death. Then, her soul further gestating, she transformed yet again. While I was learning to make jewelry, my mother entered her own cocoon without telling a soul and re-emerged spectacularly altered in her appearance and taste.

A Parallel Chrysalis

After Mitch died, Mother attended a grief group and recovered as much as one can. But they'd been together and deeply in love for seventeen years. She never met anyone else, or tried to. For the rest of her life she sometimes woke up at night and cried. "When you have a good relationship with a man," she told me, "there's nothing like it."

However, she remained fascinated by everything health-related, political, archeological and so on; and, after a dozen years on her own, her continued love for and fascination with life evolved into a wonderful sense of personal style.

She'd always worn long-waisted dresses to emphasize her own long waist and offset her excess weight. But most of these dresses were cheap polyester, too short and they ranged in general from boring, like the black with white trim, to hideous, her favorite, a garish chartreuse.

Then in Mother's last several years, despite her many pieces of honey-sweetened bread and large meals, she became seriously underweight, her ribs protruding unattractively and unhealthily. ("Isn't it ironic," she said. "After all those years of fighting my weight, I can't put on a pound!") But her new weight brought out her cheekbones and nicely shaped brown eyes framed by the gray-white hair at her temples and forehead. (In back her hair was still her natural brown. Her lipstick sometimes overshot her lips, but she'd dropped the henna years before, thus avoiding the orange hair of some elderly women.) And, clothed, she looked slender.

Taking advantage of the fact, she began to wear long, elegant-looking dresses that she purchased at thrift shops, especially the one outside her Santa Monica exercise class. She enhanced her new clothes with big dramatic costume jewelry that Mitch in his day, or me in my current bargain-hunting incarnation, found for her. (Her style did not coincide with the jewelry I knew how to make.) She mixed the costume pieces with her Mexican silver. Setting off her clothing and accessories, Mother wore the genuine leather Gaucho hat I picked up for her at a yard sale. She bragged to everyone of its provenance: from me, from a yard sale, for her. "Oh, this hat is just perfect!" she told me over and over. Its broad brim protected her face from the sun and prevented what few skin cancers such shade might afford. It also provided her new clothing style with just the right subtly sensational element for the total effect. Though increasingly stooped over her cane with scoliosis, she looked as if she'd just stepped out of a magazine for glamorous seniors.

Indeed, strangers frequently came up to her. "You're beautiful," they exclaimed. She related these experiences to me in surprise. "I look in the mirror and I just don't see it."

"I do." Just as I'd witnessed the metamorphosis of her psyche, I now noted her physical transformation. "I see it," I told her every time we visited, at least once a week.

***

Every Monday from nine in the morning until one in the afternoon, a local farmers' market set up in a parking lot five blocks from my apartment. Each Monday at noon, at the last possible moment, I rolled out of bed, threw myself into the shower, dressed, snatched up my shopping cart and lugged it, along with my body, down the street. There I selected fresh and often organic produce for Mother and me. On Monday nights she came by my apartment to pick up her share.

She was no longer able to enter my apartment. When at age seventy she had fallen in her yard taking out the trash, due to her chemotherapy-induced osteoporosis, she broke her hip. Over time the prosthetic replacement decreased her mobility even as her bones further deteriorated. This disability made it impossible for her to mount the few steps of my apartment house. So when Mother visited, she sat behind the wheel of her battered, faded (from turquoise to nearly white) 1976 Toyota station wagon, which she double-parked outside my apartment and from within which she asked what I thought of her latest apparel and matching jewelry. She always chose perfect earrings and a necklace to go with her latest thrift-shop dress. "You look fantastic," I answered honestly. Continually amazed, I delighted in the flowering of her beauty and fashion.

She accepted my acclaim more easily than that of strangers. No trace of ego accompanied that acceptance but only a hunger that grew from her own teen years, so painfully vacant of the praise she'd craved, and had deserved. In her old age she never quite believed in her beauty. But after a time she enjoyed the response her new self elicited.

After her fashion show I paraded my own newest creations for her. Learning to make jewelry, I discovered more than a new source of my own joy. I placed a few pairs of earrings on consignment in three or four stores, from the Craft and Folk Art Museum Gift Store to a boutique in Beverly Hills, sold them and bought ore beads.

Now, at my necklace of pale green jade monkeys or earrings of garnet briolettes, Mother's face grew exceptionally animated and her mouth opened in a big round "O" of pleasure and surprise.

Mothers are wonderful.

Concluding our mutual admiration society, I loaded up her trunk with the fresh produce I'd picked up for her at the market. She loved the strawberries best, during their season, delighted that they were both tastier and cheaper than those she found in supermarkets. Bargains were one of her great pleasures in life. "Oh, these are so delicious. *Delicioso!"* she emphasized each week on the phone when she got home, trying to preserve at least one of the three baskets for the next day, to savor again.

But another kind of story was also in progress, one that would end differently than did her glorious transformations.

Falling

It astounds me still, how often my mother escaped death by inches. Years before she fell in her yard, she had another fall. She'd asked Mitch to install a stainless steel bar across the top of her bedroom doorway. From this she hung upside down. This bar helped her stretch her back, to ease the pain of her then mild scoliosis. One day she failed to hook up her special boots properly and she fell.

She landed on her shoulder and was never again able to raise that arm completely. But her situation could have been worse. Had she been financially limited to the inadequate physical therapy provided by her HMO, her arm would have been totally crippled for the rest of her life. Also, of course, she could have dropped onto her head.

I told her, "I'm grateful you didn't fall on your head. If I had to tell people that you died by falling on your head when you were hanging upside down in your doorway, I couldn't have kept a straight face, and people would have thought I was a monster."

She laughed. "Anything to oblige."

Mother's next narrow escape occurred years after Mitch died. She had another fall, this one yet more momentous. Her routine at the time was this: Home from grocery shopping, she parked in the handicapped space on the gentle slope of her street. Then, one hand on her (by this time) four-pronged cane, the other on her car, she moved along the car to the trunk where, to cut down the number of trips between her car and house, she pulled out her cart and packed into it as many grocery bags as possible. Lastly, placing her cane in the cart, she leaned over, gripped the cart handle, started up the shallow rise of the street and onto the sidewalk. There she met her next obstacle, the short but steep dirt path leading from the sidewalk to her cement walkway. Up this rough incline Mother propelled her cart.

On one particular night, halfway up, she gave the cart an extra push over a little rut and discovered to her terror that she'd dangerously overloaded the cart. It stalled. She lost her balance. She started to fall backwards, toward the cement sidewalk.

Just at that exact moment, a young man was passing by. Pausing, caught by intuition in the first fractions of a second before my mother's fall became irrevocable, he asked, "Are you all right?"

I could imagine her eyes wide with fright as she replied with her perpetual courtesy. "I'm falling. Can you catch me?"

He did.

When she called to relate the story to me, we shuddered, united by horror. During the decades Mother worked, she'd typed up lawsuits brought by people crippled or killed in car accidents, not to mention more unusual accidents such as that of the woman who sat on a recently solvent-cleaned toilet seat and severely burned her buttocks. Now Mother and I, joined in that history of horror stories, imagined the agony and terror she'd have felt if she'd continued her nightmarish backward tumble onto the cement that night.

As to her rescuer, he told her he was her new neighbor but she didn't think to ask where he lived. She never saw him again. He remained another mysterious stranger, literally coming out of the night to save her and then vanish forever.

Not long after that incident, Mother had a second death-defying drama with her cart. She was unloading groceries into it when the car began to roll downhill, toward her. Somehow on her four-pronged cane, she scooted out of the way, falling as the car missed her by inches. Another neighbor saw what had happened and raced over. He chased the car, jumped in, put on the brakes before the car could hit the intersection, and returned to help Mother to her feet. That was the fall that broke her back. The next day her violent back pain began.

On yet a third night she narrowly avoided becoming a casualty from a drive-by shooting. Emerging from her car, she was heading toward her trunk at her slow, careful pace. A car pulled up. Someone inside it shot a young man less than two yards from her on her gang-ridden street. ("There aren't any gangs on *this* street," she insisted for years. "Just the streets to either side." Then one day, sheepishly, "The police shut down the little store on my corner. They were selling liquor to minors. It was a gang locus.") Had her timing been just a hair off, she might accidentally have been shot herself.

She could have died on any of those occasions. Someone, or sheer luck, always saved her. There were so many close calls in her life. But the fall in her yard when she was seventy and taking out the trash, the fall that broke her hip, would prove the mortal one.

Going Under

This morning in the yard of my mother's house I lean back in my metal chair, enveloped in the morning cold and damp. My mother survived cancer and the death of her beloved husband. Her strength and her mother's, too, run in my blood. Yet I seem unable to handle this unmodified tangle of guilt, bewilderment, shock, and mourning. How ironic if my feelings of inadequacy in the face of life, feelings I learned in my childhood, make me unable to get through the pain of the death of the now beloved person who, so long ago, inculcated these feelings in me.

But, after all, that would be only one of the ironies. There is another that I can no longer suppress, nor can I make sense of it. When Mother was eighty-six, two-and-a-half decades after she conquered cancer, all her tumors long since dissolved, there came another seemingly insuperable challenge. On Mother's small kitchen table she kept her recent disease/healing files. The latest one was for herself. She reviewed it daily. It contained the information she was collecting that might help her achieve victory once more, this time over a ruinous disease of the brain. Next to her files stood the supplements for Alzheimer's that she'd begun assembling, based on her research.

Assuming that diagnosis, so hard-won through the maze of her HMO, was correct, it's possible that healing it would have been her other, major medical miracle. But her fall in the yard, compounded by a kind of fall of my own, intervened.

Severe chronic stress, due to my neighbors' noise and hostility, activated my mysterious retrovirus, and a permanent set of illnesses broke out. The timing was deadly. The very retrovirus that had finalized healing Mother's and my relationship would hinder my ability to help her when she needed me. Indeed it would become one of the most prominent strands in the cord of calamity that closed off her life.

"You have to expect..."

My deadly stress was this: I'd lived in the same bachelor apartment for nearly thirty years. No bedroom and instead of a kitchen, I had closet-sized cooking space—my culinary cubbyhole—with a fridge and double-burner hotplate. This apartment had always been too small. But it was a quiet refuge from the noisy LA streets. I've always been sensitive to noise. Six years ago, my apartment house got new owners. They installed a new manager who loved to blast his television and stereo and who filled the building with new tenants as loud and rude as he.

Doug, in his early twenties, was the first. A musician, he moved into the single unit above me and used it as a sound studio.

"Whenever I hear him come into his apartment," I told Mother, who was as interested in the details of my life as I was in hers, "my every muscle goes rigid with tension. His stereo thunders on my ceiling. The booming bass makes my heart lose its rhythm. It roars from noon till early evening, when he finally leaves for work. He's back at 2:00 a.m., announcing himself with the slam of his door, followed by the bang of his window going up or down then the crash of his toilet seat going up or down. Then he races around with his German shepherd for five minutes. Then, wearing heavy workman boots, he and his big dog clatter down the stairs and stampede past my apartment, out the door and back ten minutes later. Since I asked him to please be more quiet, he now concludes his return with a few deafening notes from his electric guitar to let me know who's boss."

"Oh, my god. What will you do?"

"I don't know. The owners just won't help."

But I had to do something. I stopped sleeping more than a few hours a night and woke with my hands stiff with pain. After a couple of months, nodules appeared on two fingers of my right hand, a giant knot of nodules broke out on my left knee and my blood pressure shot up. I developed Chronic Fatigue Syndrome, which can cause a hypersensitivity to certain sounds and volumes, the very ones to which I was daily being subjected. In people with this super-sensitivity, a condition called hyperacusis, the brain interprets these sounds as a form of pain. The more noise Doug made, the less I slept, and the less I slept, the more painfully his noise assaulted my body.

Then there was pain as pain.

A kind of roving muscle pain commenced. It was as if I'd severely overdone exercise and my muscles ached horribly. This aching seized my neck for a few days; you don't realize the neck muscles you need to get out of bed until they hurt like that. Then the pain migrated to the left side of my ribs and, after that, to the inside of my left thigh, which was so sore I had to drag my leg along as might Dr. Frankenstein's assistant. "The building owners just tell me to call the police," I told Mother. So that's what I did. "Sometimes they catch Doug at it and tell him to be quiet. But since our apartments face the street, he usually sees them coming and gets quiet and I look like a fool. Sometimes the police are sympathetic. But a lot of times they just tell me, 'This is apartment living. You have to expect it.' I can't think of anything else to do."

"Don't those people know that literal torturers use loud noise and sleep deprivation as tools of their trade?"

"What people? My neighbors?"

"The landlord!"

"Either they don't believe me—it's a couple—or they don't care."

The rheumatologist I saw informed me, "You have fibromyalgia, which is causing your muscle pain. You also have Synovitis." This was an inflammation in my joints. The doctor explained that when a joint became swollen, red and hot, the disease was eating up my connective tissue. He recommended I take non-steroidal anti-inflammatories and gave me a prescription. "You need to take them at the highest dose every day."

But Mother gave me the holistic medicine journals to which she still subscribed. They stated that every chronic disease, including mine, was systemic, and that non-steroidal anti-inflammatories just hide the symptoms and ultimately weaken your whole body.

Yet my stress persisted and my pain escalated. Both my hands became so painfully inflamed I had to open doors with my elbows and lick the food off my plate because pain made holding silverware too excruciating.

"What do you think I should do?" I asked my mother.

"I don't know," she admitted.

After three weeks I was ready to give up and fill the doctor's prescription. This was during the O.J. trial. The day before I took my prescription to the drug store, one of the O.J. jurors had to go to the hospital. She'd had a bad reaction to her non-steroidal anti-inflammatories.

I thought, *Uh-oh.*

I continued researching. Naturally, it was Mother who found the solution. A single supplement brought my inflammation under control for the next few years. But another problem surfaced. One year of sleeplessness and noise-induced stress caused my whole immune system to crash.

Crash

Without warning my white cells, red cells, hematocrit, hemoglobin and platelets plummeted. My old AIDS fright came back, whipping adrenalin through my veins. The lowest normal reading for white cells, the reading I'd had since the ozone, was four thousand. Within three months they dropped to twenty-eight hundred. My platelets went from two hundred sixty to one hundred forty-five, still clearly on their way down. When I went to my HMO doctor, she said, "We should think about a bone marrow test. We don't know what's going on."

No, I thought, recalling the agony in Mother's widening eyes when she'd had a bone marrow test. *We really shouldn't think about that.* Growing fear ignited the low-grade fever that had persisted for ten years after the ozone treatment and periodically returned. That night I lay on my bed and told myself aloud, quietly, over and over, with as much force as I could muster, "This isn't AIDS. I can handle whatever it is. My mother had *terminal cancer.* My mother came back from the dead. So can I."

"Of course you can," Mother encouraged when I shared my mantra. "I know you can do it."

Committing myself to that feat, I put myself on a 24-hour a day holistic program. I did acupuncture; healing energy meditations; and, like Mother, I took coffee enemas (with a normal-sized tube) at one end of my body while, into the other, I dropped massive amounts of supplements. A friend I'd made at a health food store decades earlier loaned me money for this round of survival supplements.

I also resorted to juicing.

I ran enough veggies through my juicer to make sixty ounces of juice per day. The amount of produce necessary for this output was staggering. I covered that expense by trading earrings I made to a farmer at the local open market.

Juicing was just as labor-intensive, time-consuming and exhausting as I'd imagined when I observed Mother doing it during her cancer. Now addressing her with irony, I paraphrased a line from an existential movie I saw in the sixties. "Am I juicing to live or living to juice?"

Mother laughed. She hadn't seen the movie. But she got the meaning and loved the linguistic play of the line.

However, my survival program was tedious, leaving me no time for writing, and this was increasingly depressing. Not only did I love to write. It remained the one thing that gave me a feeling of power over my life. One day I would get the skill thing right. I had important stories to tell and writing was still my sole, if merely potential, vehicle to autonomy, not to mention solvency. I had to pay back my mother and my friend for their financial assistance. I didn't want to end up on someone's floor sorting pennies.

I obsessed over my blood counts as feverishly as during my AIDS years. After a month I returned to Suzann's clinic for blood tests. My numbers had stopped falling and instead were creeping back up. I nearly keeled over with relief and gratitude toward everyone who'd helped, especially Mother, whose encouragement I welcomed unambiguously. In three months I got all my blood counts back to low normal—in the view of my conventional doctor, they came back up "as spontaneously" as they'd dropped.

Immediately, I cut back on my acupuncture trips, pills, meditation time; and I stopped juicing altogether. I wanted to rescue my quality of life, such as it was.

My second immune crash, six years after the first, occurred just months before Mother's hip surgery. If I hadn't gotten the message the first time, I got it then.

Each of my successive overhead fellow tenants kept similar hours, announcing their two a.m. arrivals by making similar banging, explosive sounds. But, worse, their loud stereos and televisions never ceased reverberating through my ceiling and walls, flesh and bones. Bass thunder sent me ricocheting off my walls as well as the walls in the apartment corridor, for loud tenants inhabited the entire building.

"What is it with all these guys with their sense of entitlement to make noise?" I demanded of Mother rhetorically. "My most courteous Good Little Girl request for a little quiet brings out a hostility in them that borders on the pathological."

"Oh, I feel so terrible for you!"

Moreover, the apartment manager, who hated me because I did not share his love of loudness, brought in young, manipulable tenants. He promoted not only their noise but their antagonism toward me. They laughed at or ignored me whenever I asked them to please turn down their whatever, and they nuked me with glances of such enmity when they passed me in the hallway that their attitude made me nearly as ill as did the noise.

Like the first time, my white count and other blood values started dropping. I was a little less frightened than when it happened before. *I brought myself back to normal last time*, I told myself. *I can do it again.* And, by the same methods as before, I did return to "borderline normal." But in addition to the fact that my immune system was still functioning at only half my own normal—half of what I'd had before the virus and the ozone treatment—my return from this second crash was taking longer than during the previous episode. I noticed with stark clarity that there was no guarantee I could keep stabilizing myself. My unknown virus would always underlie my health status. The cancers associated with all known retroviruses endangered me. Stress could always produce potentially life-threatening crises.

I couldn't afford to keep living in that apartment.

But I also couldn't afford to move.

A Battle

Despising the idea of spending my meager energy hunting for a new apartment, I'd put it off until now, telling myself the next tenant would be quieter and courteous. But, finally recovered from my crash, I had to acknowledge that my living situation was never going to improve. I had to get out of there.

Thus I discovered the housing crisis. Rents had shot through the hole in the ozone. While I'd procrastinated looking, developers and management companies had taken over the city. A living space with only four electrical outlets and a room half the size of mine cost a hundred dollars more a month than I was paying, or could pay. I did find one landlady who charged $500 a month for a one-bedroom; I was paying that for my bachelor. But of course she had no vacancies, and as there were only eight units in her building, I could not picture anyone ever moving out. However, she said she was putting me at the top of her list should a unit ever become available. I said I'd call her once a month just in case.

I looked for a month-and-a-half after my second crash ended. I looked until Mother went into the hospital for her surgery. Antagonism had surrounded me for years, noise bombarding me remorselessly. I'd acquired a permanent insomnia which left me walking around in a stupor of exhaustion with flensed nerves, jumping blood pressure, migrating muscle pain, joint pain, and on the verge of a scream of rage and despair that went on in my head all the time. I'd also developed more deformities in my hands, wrists and toes, and a new rheumatologist rediagnosed my Synovitis as Undifferentiated Connective Tissue Disease (and would later re-diagnose it again, as Rheumatoid Arthritis). I'd lost three teeth with more threatened because I clenched what teeth remained during what sleep I got; and whatever gray cells could still carry thought moved along like drunken slugs through molasses.

But Mother's brain cells were in worse shape. She'd been forgetting things for a few years. While in the past I'd called her several times a week for reassurance for myself, now in a role reversal I was calling her several times a day to make sure she was all right.

Then, a year before her surgery, she began to exhibit small moments of dementia.

Recalling landslide of events that began at that time—her severe mental slippage and apparent recovery, her hip operation and what followed—I battle falling into that chasm of such severe depression that I can imagine no return.

***

A month-and-a-half after I started looking for an apartment, Mother entered the nursing care system and I quit looking.

A Good Life

For three years prior to her hip operation, Mother had asserted to me that she needed the surgery. But each time she came back from seeing the orthopedic surgeon, she proclaimed, "I can't do this *now!* There's so much to do *first.*"

She wanted to find a place for the boxes of supplements that lay atop the masses of one-pound bags of herbs that covered the bed in the small, spare bedroom that once had been mine and then belonged to Mitch. She also wanted to bring some order to her files, which were in extreme disarray. She wanted to put her house in order either to come back to after the surgery or so that I wouldn't have to deal with it if she died during thc operation. "I can't die now," she insisted. "I'd be embarrassed to have you deal with all this!"

On the other hand she'd expressed many times the desire to die before Alzheimer's, or whatever caused her symptoms, destroyed her mind. "Intellectual pursuits have been my greatest joy in life," she told me as well as her regular HMO physician, Dr. Burns. She loved life but on her terms. "If I don't have quality of life, if I don't have my mind, I don't have anything."

She was also terrified she might outlive her small nest egg. Even if she discovered the key to reversing her Alzheimer's symptoms—or, if the Alzheimer's diagnosis was wrong, if she eliminated whatever else was destroying her brain—she dreaded the prospect of living on her Social Security alone.

She wanted the freedom to buy books, subscribe to magazines, contribute to causes in which she believed, replace machines that broke. Most of all a life of quality for my mother came down to her health. The only pharmaceutical she took was thyroid medication; very unusual for an elderly person in our culture. Doctors put most elderly people on six or seven drugs, some to counteract the side effects of others. Most of them cause one problem or another. Mother's health was far from perfect. But if she could no longer afford her numerous supplements, healthy eating habits and the odd machine she purchased, she was certain the health she did enjoy, mental and physical, would swiftly deteriorate.

Seniors comprise thirteen percent of the population but twenty percent of the suicides. If Mother's money ran out or she failed to find an answer to her waning mental acuity, she planned to join them. Investigating the Hemlock Society, she told me, "I want you to get their book on suicide."

"Okay." I got both the book and tape. But although I shared her quality-of-life attitude, I found her suicidal statements ghoulish. "I'm going to put a plastic bag over my head when the time comes," she kept saying.

"Well, the Hemlock Society recommends a kind of gas you can get at K-Mart to ease the stress of dying like that." Always trying to be helpful. But I never got it for her. I harbored horrid pictures of walking into her bedroom and finding her wearing a plastic bag on her head, her face contorted with terror or pain, the suicide somehow gone wrong.

But I said nothing of this. Her plastic bag lay some distance in the future. It might never happen. She made no effort, other than getting the book, to make it real. Why fuel that goal? After all, she could die on the operating table.

The time came when she could no longer postpone her surgery. She set a date. "Don't feel bad if I die." Still spreading pillows around me. "I don't mind. I've had a good life." And then there came the glimmer that stupefied us. Changes in her memory made it suddenly seem possible that she was about to rescue herself from her mental losses. If so, and if she survived the hip operation, she could return home, walk again without pain—and think clearly once more. Despite its imperfections, her good life might continue for a few, or several, more years... Could she have done it?

Inner Smile

I think about what Mother learned in order to triumph over a "fatal" cancer, and of the physical processes and products I learned about from her and implemented to save my own life from my retrovirus. But I still struggle to make her psychological revolution my own. What would *she* have done to survive this dark, unshakable weight of tears, were our situations reversed? How do I change down to my own roots?

Before Mother's operation I made time to see my psychologist a few times. She told me that the latest studies indicate that all journeys through traumatic memories should be accompanied by positive thoughts or good feelings. "All the latest clinical studies say you need to have a positive base when you're going through the process of healing pain," she said. "You need a happy memory or maybe a loving image."

This concept coincides with the spirituality I inadequately practice.

Building on my previous energy work, I saw a qi gong master last year. He started each session of physical exercises by having me meditate on happiness. "Qi" means "energy." Qi gong, an ancient Chinese discipline, teaches the cultivation and balance of energy. During my lessons we would stand opposite each other. Master Zhou would say, "Energy flow better with happy feeling." He would grin, gesturing down his body with a hand, indicating the flow of qi. "Happy thoughts!"

My friend Marcia teaches another system of Chinese healing meditations. In the first one I learned from her, she taught me to circulate "the inner smile," a kind of smiling energy, through different parts of my body.

Then there's acupuncture, which also balances your energy. One acupuncturist told me, "The body has an intelligence that has nothing to do with the brain." Balance enables that body intelligence to manifest itself, as health.

I remember all this now, and I think that energy itself has intelligence. I don't believe in the Judeo-Christian versions of the divine. But from Eastern disciplines to modern psychology, the intelligence of the universe appears to be an impulse toward wellness; and intrinsic to wellness is joy; and to joy, love.

I once read about a study where blood tests were taken before and after people watched a film about Mother Teresa. Test results after the film showed an increase in the subjects' immune function. In addition, more than one medical study shows that people who have a loving relationship, if only with a pet, raise their immunity to disease. So even Western medicine, objective physical science, with its material emphasis, dictates that the impulse of life, the divine impulse, is toward health, and that love, compassion, and kindness are integral to it.

And I believe this, too, I always have. But only theoretically. I haven't done the actual work. I haven't dug my roots deeply enough into my qi gong practice, my healing meditations or my psychological journeys to center myself in faith in that divine impulse.

Yet without that faith, where do you find in the death of a loved one, especially an awful and unnecessary death, a way to accept and transcend what happened? I want to find in my soul that which can honor the reality of what my mother underwent, and my own bleak journey with her, and yet not become mired forever in that hell.

So I need to focus on the positive, the happy thought—the love that grew between us steadily during the quarter century following her cancer.

And I must remember that as part of her own transformation, my mother met another overpowering health challenge with courageous determination. She overcame monsters and fought through to a second victory. I have to remember that so long as she could live in her house and had her autonomy, to whatever degree she could still ambulate, drive, think, read and laugh, she triumphed, despite everything, miraculously.

But even as I search for a remnant of Mother's legacy within myself, her special gift of transcendence and triumph, panic continues to wrench my heart and sorrow keens through my blood. My mother's final victory, achieved through phenomenal effort, returns to me. But always at the back of my mind, running through those memories, as I struggle to get free of this leaden and ruthless grief which has fallen on me like a mountain, I think about fate.

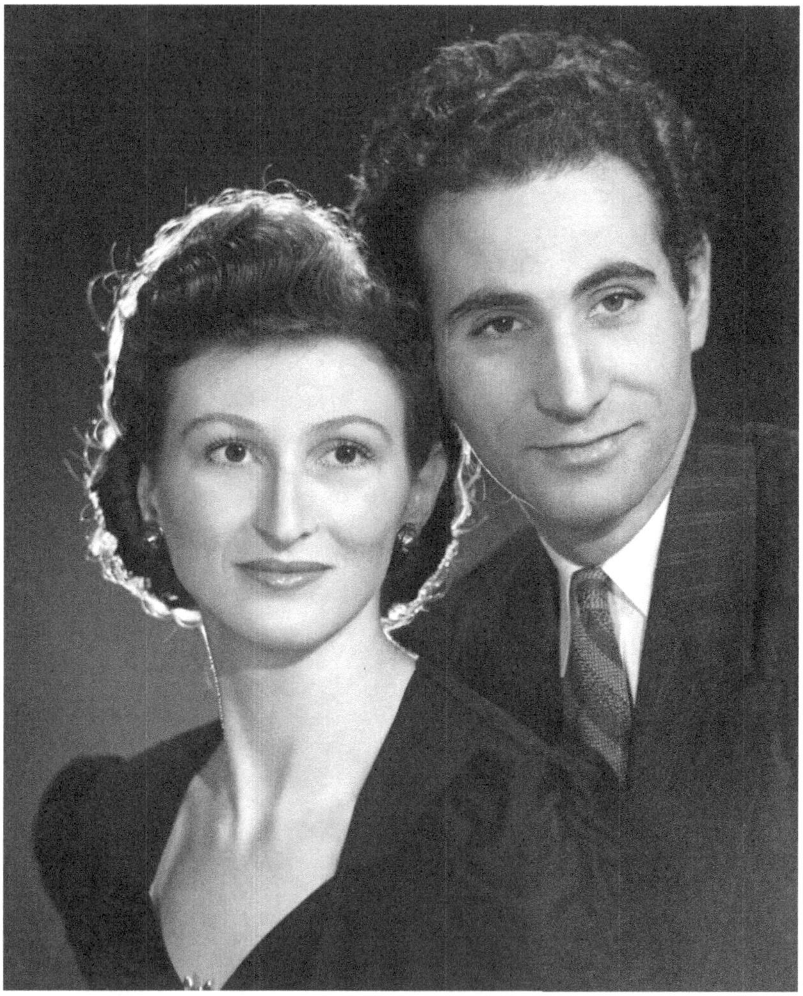

My mother and father

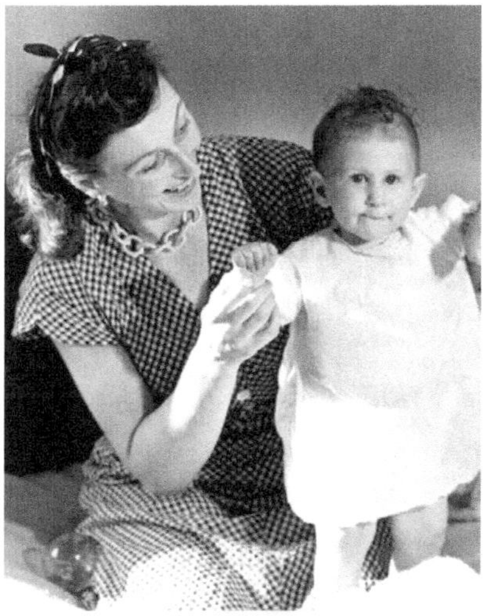

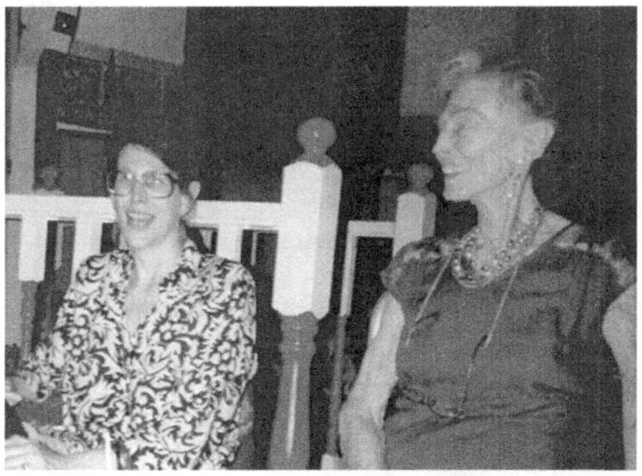

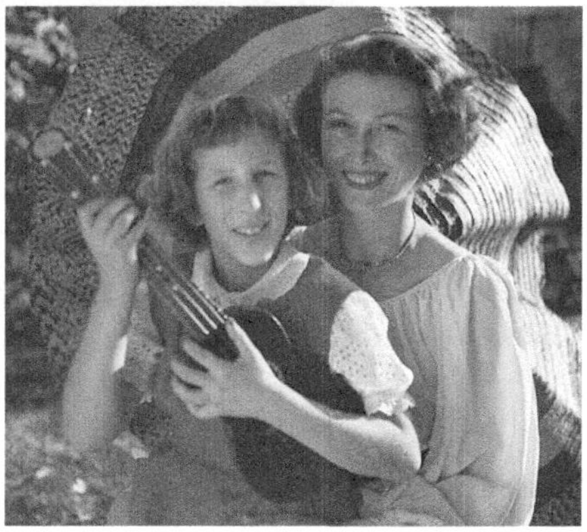

Mother and me, left to right: the young mother and infant;
Mother (at eighty-three) and me at Suzann's birthday party;
Mother and me when I had my "Dumbo" nose

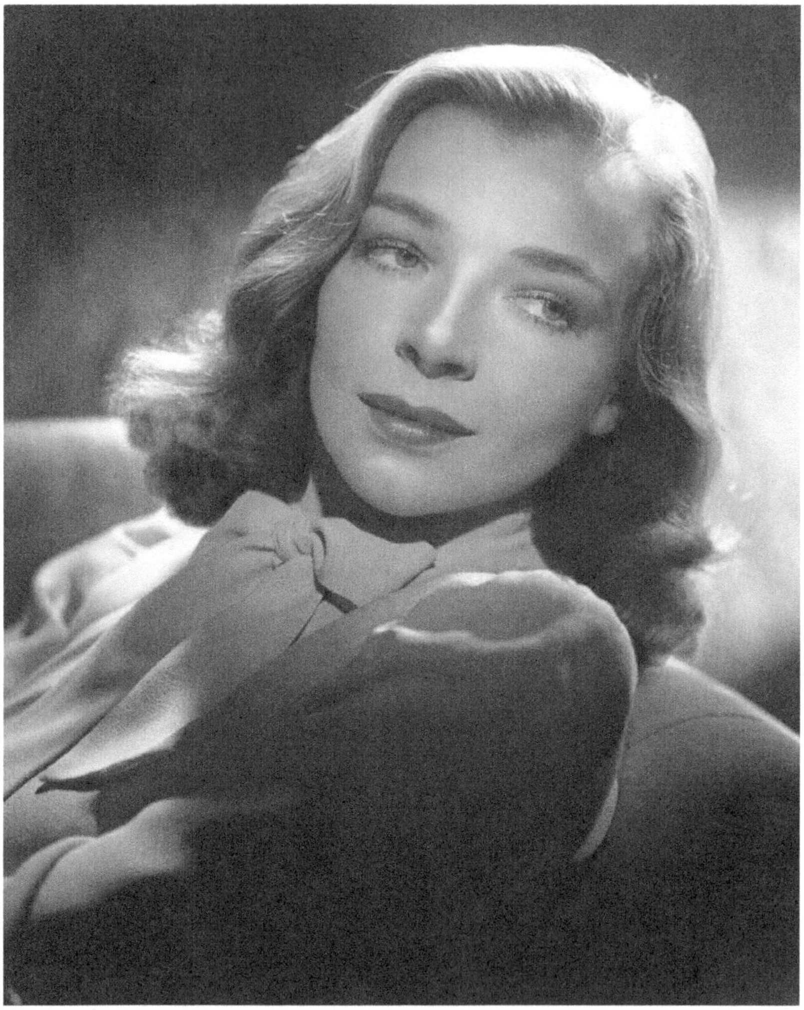

Aunt Lucy

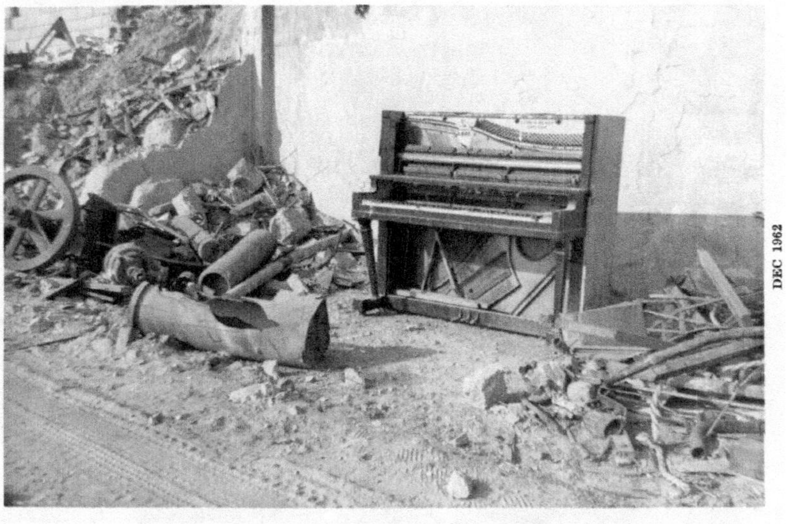

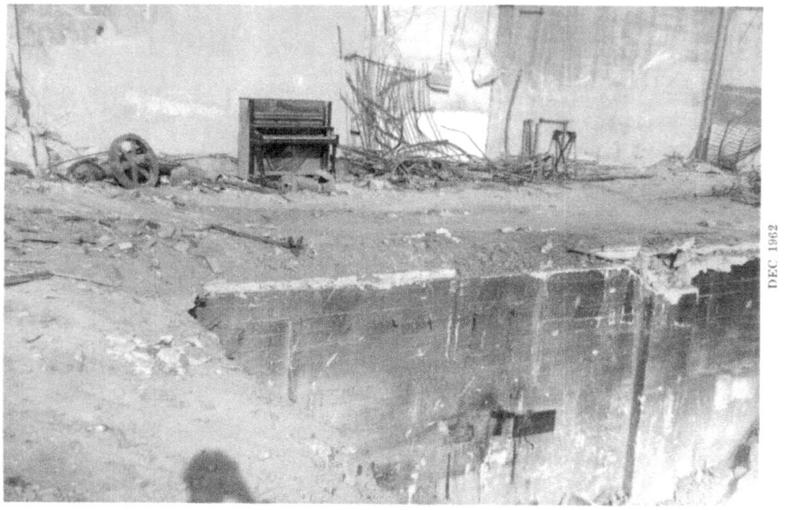

Mother's fascination with photography—
The Piano at the End of the World

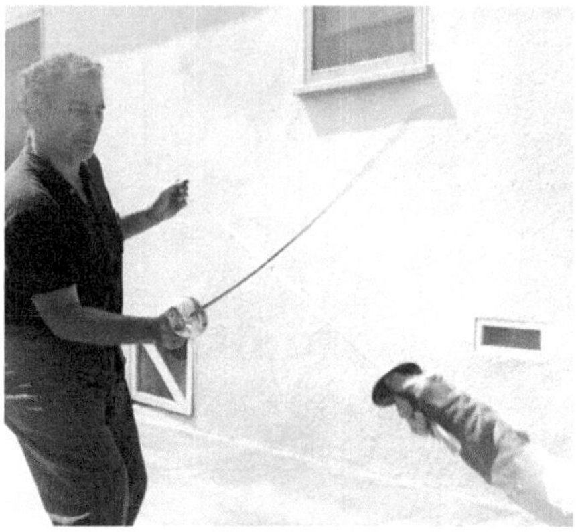

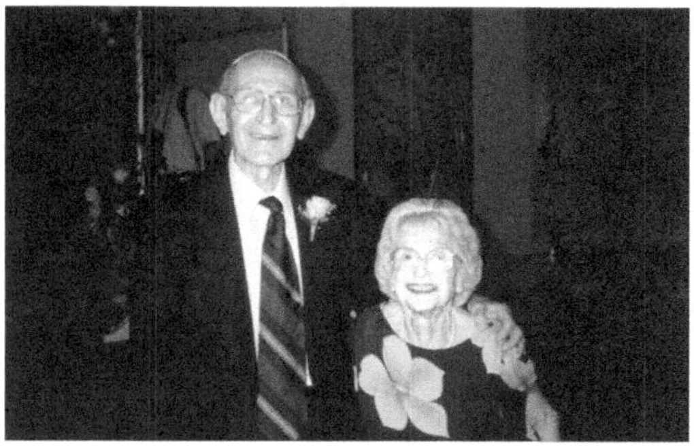

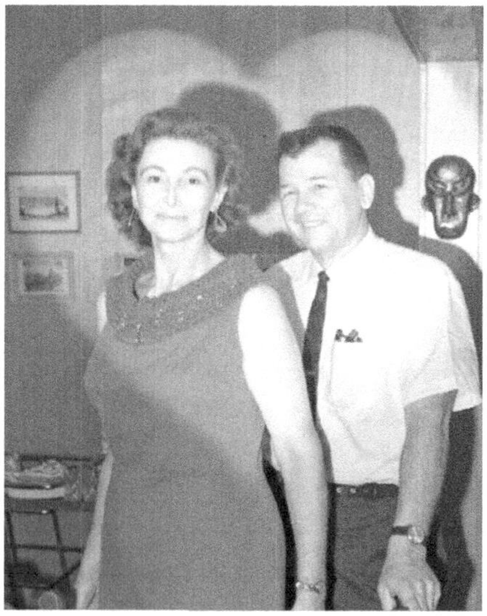

Left to right: My father teaching fencing;
Aunt Grace and Uncle Sid;
Mother and Mitch

Book Four

Last Miracle

1997 to 2000

First Incident

"I just had it in my hand!" Always lauded and amazed by friends for her excellent memory (quoting poems, lines from movies, decades-ago events), Mother grew increasingly aggravated at losing words and names, while mislaid items sent her off on long, obsessive searches. She abandoned a relaxing afternoon sitting on her deck with the birds chirping nearby, her newspaper, tea and food before her, instead to spend febrile hours rooting through the house in search of the latest lost object, however inconsequential. As she skipped one meal and then another, afternoon wheeled into later afternoon. Suddenly it was early evening. "I haven't done a goddam thing today," she told me almost daily. "I can't stand this!" At which point she would finally sit down, eat and read for the next several hours, repeating her refrain at two in the morning. "I haven't done...!"

A few years into her mental lapses, there transpired the first incident of mild dementia of which I was aware. She was eighty-four. "Where did I put that twenty-dollar bill I set aside for the gardener? I think I'm losing my mind!" A mere expression of frustration. Or was it? By accident she found the twenty. She'd taped it to the bottom of a honey jar on the kitchen table.

"Why would you tape money to the bottom of a honey jar?" I laughed, although I was uneasy. It was a really weird thing to do. Yet what triggered my anxiety was less the act than her defense of it.

She did not laugh back. "I'm sure I had a very good reason." Her voice held no trace of the humor or irony that would have been her customary response under such circumstances. Her voice instead expressed denial.

The previous year she'd taken a labyrinthine safari through her HMO to learn what exactly was causing her worsening memory. The trek was arduous and obtained neither information nor diagnosis. In fact it was a farce. We let the whole subject go. But this episode compelled me to call the Alzheimer's Association, where I discovered in the literature they sent that denial is a symptom of Alzheimer's.

But how do you know what kind of denial you're dealing with? Denial had always been part of my mother's personality. "Oh, I just don't believe that!" she'd said all my life of anything that failed to conform to whatever belief, expectation or desire she already possessed, including in my childhood and teens when she denied my feelings and bad experiences, which were not life, just dress rehearsals.

In the last several years, whenever she was sick, her denial made me crazy on her behalf rather than mine.

"I'm okay," she'd say. "I'll be okay." "I'm sure I'll be better tomorrow." "I'm sure this isn't anything." This denial allowed her to avoid a trip to the doctor. "This isn't a serious cough." Then I listened on the phone as she interrupted herself, or me if I was speaking, at every other syllable, with a deep, rumbling, volcanic cough that erupted in her chest, convulsing her for several minutes. When it finished, we further paused while I listened to her forcibly heaving up vast coagulations of phlegm. Then she announced with cheerful authority, "I'm fine."

"You sound like you're hacking up Atlantis."

"Oh, I'd know a serious cough."

Eventually, she'd have to go to the doctor, who almost invariably pronounced her condition as pneumonia and/or bronchitis. She'd had pneumonia as a young woman and her lungs remained susceptible.

But when denial occurs in people with Alzheimer's and other particular conditions of actual brain damage like schizophrenia, the individuals are literally incapable of perceiving reality accurately. Had this become the case? But how was I to differentiate her normal denial from Alzheimer's?

To further complicate Mother's situation, a breakdown of the brain doesn't happen all at once, at least with Alzheimer's. My friend Ruthie's mother had

Alzheimer's. When she, the mother, was in the early stages of the disease, she gathered her children about her one night and said, "There's something wrong. I'm forgetting things."

Ruthie and her sister reassured their mother. "Everyone forgets things."

"But she knew," Ruthie told me. "She said, 'No. This is different. There's something wrong.'" In the beginning, Ruthie's mother knew. Later, she didn't.

My mother too sometimes recognized that something was wrong. But she rejected her awareness of it in the next conversation, or moment. Or she might admit a particular behavior was inexplicable but refuse to accept Alzheimer's or another form of senile dementia as the explanation.

Yet, *was* something really wrong? Or was this just Mother, her absent-minded and in-denial self exaggerated by age? The incidents of bizarre behavior accrued. But when I tried to talk to my family about it, they rejected—they denied—what I was seeing.

Over and over I told both of my aunts, Lucy and Grace, and my Uncle Sid, how worried I was becoming about Mother; they, all in her same age group, kept responding, "Oh, I do that, too." Like Ruthie's children. *Everyone forgets things.*

"No, you don't," I insisted with growing anxiety. I described incidents in detail. My mother's denial isolated me from her. I didn't want my few relatives' denial to isolate me from them, too. I didn't want to be alone with my mother's failing mind. Yet I could see their point.

The behaviors I described to them were in fact similar to those of their own aging selves. Moreover, despite the extreme irrationality of some of Mother's acts, those incidents were still quite rare; and in the same period that they occurred, her old acumen clung on, further masking the aberrant moments. Anyone who wasn't talking to her several times a day, as I did, would be confused by my fears.

In fact, I, too, sometimes had trouble accepting Mother's mental anomalies as real. Maybe *I* was imagining things. Maybe I *was* wrong. For, with the same spunk and stubbornness that helped her overcome “terminal” cancer, Mother’s intelligence, undeterred by memory shortfalls, helped her meet the predators of the elderly.

One time that intelligence saved her money. A second time it might have saved her life. But then it too foundered before the assault of Alzheimer’s.

Challenges

A young man and woman approached Mother in a local grocery store. They claimed to have grown up on her street, a one-block horseshoe that forms a cozy neighborhood all its own. "I don't remember them," Mother confided to me. Actually, she didn't remember most of the multitude of children, now grown up, whom she and Mitch had befriended over the decades. But she was "pleased and warmed" by their concern for her as the three renewed their acquaintance. "It's quite wonderful."

A few weeks later she told me, "They want to hide some of their money in my credit card account."

"That sounds very suspicious. Don't do it."

"I'll find out more." She found out the next week. Disillusion and disgust tinged her voice. "They just wanted to get my credit card number."

The next year a far more dangerous couple attempted to make Mother their prey. "They followed me home. They told me I'd hit someone at Sunset and Echo Park and that I shouldn't call the police."

"Oh, my god."

The month before, after a lifetime with a perfect driving record, Mother was pulling into a parking lot when another car broad-sided her. The other car was only going five miles an hour, barely denting her door. "I wasn't doing anything wrong!" my mother proclaimed. But the driver insisted, and a witness confirmed, that she was at fault. I hadn't doubted it. I'd witnessed enough myself to become leery of driving with her, although I hadn't stopped.

Whenever she was in my neighborhood, Mother took me on several errands. A couple of hours with her saved me four or five days on the bus. We also made the occasional long distance trip together, like into Van Nuys to see an excellent chiropractor. But I was noticing that my mother's reflexes on the road had slowed and she became more easily befuddled than in the past.

Yet this so-called accident, as described by her new acquaintances, sounded all wrong. "They said you *shouldn't* call the police? Why would anyone urge you *not to call the police?"*

"I don't know. They wanted to use my bathroom."

"Oh, no."

"I had to let them into the house."

"You didn't!" My well-mannered mother, smiling, no doubt, the while.

"Then they wanted me to go back with them to where the accident happened, to show me. They kept asking me to ride back with them in their truck."

Apprehension made me queasy. "And?"

"I was polite but I insisted on following them back in my car."

"Good for you," I exploded in relief. My ever-intelligent mother, not as naive or passive as I'd thought. "Then what happened?"

"I followed them. We didn't see anything. No police. There was no evidence of any accident."

"If they contact you again, if they call or knock, don't answer. Whatever you do, *don't let them in."*

"Don't worry, I won't!"

I was very nervous for her for the next month. They knew she lived alone, and where. But they never came back. Whatever they'd planned for her, it involved having her alone in their truck. She'd been savvy enough to avoid that. But the next year a man got her phone number from the Internet. He also got her age and tried to take advantage of it to inveigle her into an investment scheme. He nearly got her.

"Inflation is going to eat up your savings," he warned, "and you could get caught by medical expenses that'll wipe you out."

She knew that. Her dwindling nest egg had already heightened her lifelong fear of poverty. Now this man boosted her fear to a new plateau, deliberately setting her up then following the set-up with his investment "solution." She told me, "It's 12% guaranteed interest."

Could she actually be considering this? "You know there's nothing safe that's 12% interest."

"Yes, I know," she admitted reluctantly.

But my relief hovered uncertainly. There was something in her tone. "What does he say it's for?"

"Commercial paper."

"But you won't do it?"

She stalled.

"Don't even consider it."

More silence. An obstinate silence! My stomach did a little flip. Alarm gripped me. At no time in her life would she have done other than bluntly reject the deal.

"I'll have to learn more about it."

"There's nothing more to learn," I declared.

"I'm only thinking about investing five thousand dollars."

Apprehension gripped me. "You *know* it's a scam."

Mother reverted again to silence, sulky now, her resolve hardening.

"You can't do it!" Of all times for her stubbornness to assert itself! She'd possessed such clarity only the previous year with the couple and their truck. But now, while with one part of her mind she distinctly recognized what was going on, simultaneously she wanted so desperately to believe someone could save her from poverty that she was falling for an obvious lie. My anger against the con man added to my agitation. This man was transforming *my mother* into the cliché of the frightened old woman who grasps at irrational straws and gets taken for everything.

My fear for her was also growing on another front. "Impaired judgment" came on that list of Alzheimer's symptoms.

"Well," Mother circumlocuted. "We'll see."

See, nothing. I pulled out the heavy guns. I called Aunt Grace and Uncle Sid. Grace loved my mother as if she were her own sister. But, as I knew from being on the occasional receiving end myself, love never gave Grace the impetus for tact when she was concerned about one of us. ("I know I have a temper," she chuckles when not in the throes of it.)

I could imagine Grace haranguing my poor mother on the phone from the desert where she and Sid lived. "Are you crazy? Don't you know you can't get that kind of interest on a legitimate deal? What's the matter with you? You'll never get that money back!" Grace would have rampaged in that vein without a breath, repeating everything my mother already knew to be true about such an "investment." Then Uncle Sid would have added his own disgust. "Why don't you just give him the five thousand and be done with it?"

Mother backed down, more intimidated by us than impaired in her judgment of the con man. But there was definitely something wrong with her mind. What would become of her as it progressed?

My next experiences with her on the road indicated the grim impediments ahead.

Driving

One afternoon as we were backing out of a parking space in a lot, I saw a car and Mother did not. It was coming our way and not stopping. “Look out!” I shouted. Mother slammed on the brakes.

“It was in my blind spot,” she informed me as we sat there and the car rolled past.

“You have a blind spot the size of a big car.” Then I ventured, “Maybe you should think about giving up driving.”

She laughed.

Nor, it must be said, did I immediately cease riding with her and revert to bus trips. But one evening as she was taking me home from Trader Joe’s, her driving disability took a qualitative jump. We’d just left the parking lot and were heading up the street to my apartment when a light sprinkle began to fall. As the diminutive droplets spread over her windshield, Mother felt around the dashboard. Then, her brows bunched with anxiety, she pulled over to the curb.

“What’s wrong?” I asked, the night dark around us. “Why don’t you turn on the windshield wipers?”

“I can’t remember how. I can’t seem to find the—knob. Switch. The—” She was having trouble even finding the word. “Just give me a minute.” She thought hard, her anxiety mounting. She felt all around the dashboard again then sat still. Then she reached out and turned on the windshield wipers.

This was more than any age-related slowing of reflexes or tendency to become confused. A yawning fissure had opened, if only temporarily, in her mind.

Okay, I told myself as we continued forward, it’s time for me to stop riding with her. At least, no more shared journeys to fabulous but distant chiropractors! Climbing out of her car at my apartment, I urged her, “You really need to think about giving up driving.”

"Yes, dear, I'll think about it. When the time comes."

"The time has come. Suppose you'd forgotten how to turn on the windshield wipers on a street where you couldn't pull over?"

"That wouldn't happen."

"Why not?"

"It just couldn't!"

But a few weeks later, she stopped by on a Monday evening to pick up the produce I'd gotten for her earlier at the farmers' market. We performed our joyful fashion rituals. Then, heading home, she started down the street, her trunk filled with produce and her antediluvian faded wreck of a station wagon clanking, jumping, rattling and putt-putting loudly, her brake lights still blinking.

With a boost of adrenalin I raced down the street. Panting, I caught up with her at the corner where she'd come to a stop; she now needed about three miles leeway from oncoming traffic on either side to make a turn. I tapped urgently on the passenger window. She turned to me, her face pinched with stress.

"Your brake lights are still on."

"I know they're on!" she retorted. She'd been trying to turn them off. "I can't find the damn switch! I thought it was over here, but this doesn't seem to do anything…" She drove on, the car giving a sharp jerk every yard or two. With sadness and a slight nausea that would become familiar to me, I watched her rattle off into the night, the car jumping and jolting every few feet, the brake lights blinking. She admitted later she'd been unable to turn them off the entire way home.

The next morning her memory came back. She knew what to do.

I renewed my attempts to convince her to think about giving up her car. "You might forget something vital while you're driving and couldn't pull over."

"I won't." Stubborn as ever.

"But what if you do? You forgot where the windshield wipers are. You forgot how to turn off the brake lights. You could forget how to hit the damn brakes."

"I'd rather be dead than quit driving." A tad less courteous than usual.

Rita had politely declined Mother's invitation to drive her home from my most recent birthday party (after having accepted that same invitation the previous year and gained her own experience of Mother's driving). Now she reprised what she'd told me a few times already. "You need to get her off the road."

"Easier said than done."

"When my uncle got Alzheimer's," Rita said, "my mother anonymously wrote to the DMV and got his license revoked."

"I can't do that. If Mother ever found out, she'd feel betrayed. She would be devastated." It would destroy the relationship we'd rebuilt with love and trust for more than two decades. "There has to be something else."

Eventually I convinced Mother to stay off the freeways most of the time. But her health conventions were too complicated a drive for her to travel to on surface streets, and her weekly Santa Monica exercise class was too far. As for me, I continued to let her help me on shorter trips and saw no more dangerous incidents.

In fact at times I doubted Rita's and my perception of the urgency of the problem. Mother would drive long distances, get lost, get where she was going and get home. She'd go out, get caught in the rain, the streets slick and other drivers incompetent, and still she'd get home. Maybe I was overreacting. I stopped pushing Mother to quit driving.

Then the most shocking incident occurred. After that I concluded that driving with my mother even on local errands was too dicey.

This was the episode that frightened even her.

The Garage Episode

She was steering into her HMO garage. "I was just reaching for the ticket when, all of a sudden, the car shot forward. I was scared to death." Telling me on the phone that night, she was still shaking.

"How did it happen?" I fought the storm of anxiety that seized me.

"I don't know. The car just accelerated."

"Do you think you did something, or was it the car?"

"I was reaching for the ticket. I think—I don't know if I was still moving. I'm not sure. I keep going over it in my mind, but I just can't remember that moment. I've tried and tried."

Sickened by the possibility that my worst fears for her were coming true, I asked, "What did you do then?"

"I somehow managed to navigate the car into a chain."

"A chain? What do you mean?"

She surprised me. "I didn't know if there was anyone in the garage and I didn't want to hit another car or the garage wall. The chain stopped the car." She'd had the wit to take this action on the moment. "But I just don't know what happened."

But that was, finally, the important thing. What happened?

Walter, her mechanic, couldn't find anything wrong with her car when she took it to him the next day. Yet the vehicle did have enough age on it to have passed as a covered wagon. Walter told her, in his deep, gravelly voice, "I can't say for certain it wasn't the car." So maybe it was a once in a lifetime uncontrolled automobile launch.

But what if it was my mother? What if she did something? With astonishing presence of mind she'd directed her car into the chain and away from other people, cars and any danger to herself from hitting the wall. Yet at the same time she couldn't remember what happened just before the car surged.

A few days later she told me, "As I was sitting there today about to start the car, I could see how my foot might have slipped over the accelerator and caught under the brake."

"Do you think that's what happened?"

"I almost did it today. I can see how I might have done it. But I still can't remember anything." She would never be sure, or get over it. "I used to love driving. Now every time I get in the car I'm terrified. I have to sit there for five minutes before I can get my courage up to start it."

"And yet," I complained to Rita, "she still refuses to give up driving. Even her mechanic told her she should think about quitting driving. I talked to him. He told me. But she says she doesn't remember him saying that. She denies it."

"You have to stop her." Rita repeated her suggestion that I notify the DMV. But I just couldn't risk Mother finding out. I had to convince her to stop voluntarily.

I ranted, "What will you forget next?" For decades, including those of my formative years, Mother typed accident lawsuits and conveyed to me what she learned: a vigilance toward other drivers equal to an ancient hunter's respect for predatory, carnivorous game. She also taught me about safe driving by her own good example. She never took her eyes from the road for more than a split second. "Even one second of lost attention on the road could be fatal." I remain to this day deathly afraid of driving with anyone who dares more than the most fleeting glance at me except when at a full stop. Now I told her, "You could become distracted while you're driving in ways you didn't used to become distracted. Anything could happen."

"I don't care if I die. I'd rather die than live without a car."

"I'm not worried about your dying. That's your choice. I know you don't care if you die. But what if you injure yourself horribly and still live, or you kill or cripple someone else, like a child?"

"I wouldn't."

"You can't predict that!"

On the other hand, she had a few points on her side.

"Just think about it," she snapped back. "I have to drive. How could I shop without a car? How would I visit you? How would I go to the bank or the doctor or run up the street to the drugstore or post office?"

How *would* she survive? She was too fragile for the bus; she couldn't even mount the steps to my apartment. When she walked she had to watch every step lest she fall. Yet she couldn't afford cab fare for all the places she'd have to go for the rest of her life. "I'm fine!"

I had to find a way to help her.

***

In the past on rare occasion I'd reviewed my original decision not to learn to drive until I could afford a car. I'd also never bothered to learn because of a secret fear: that at the precise moment of a potential collision or running someone over, I would precipitate calamity myself by not trusting my instincts.

My initial resolution had been easy. When I was younger I could handle the buses. They and I were both in better shape. Over the years I'd continued to conclude I was making the right, if inconvenient, choice, not realizing I was losing the ability to choose: Every year LA grew less the place to start driving, especially for someone whose brain cells are becalmed in a Sargasso swamp of fatigue. But I never dreamed that the inconvenience of bussing would become incapacitating—or that my inability to drive would affect my mother, let alone to the extent that began to reveal itself.

I decided to find answers to Mother's questions. What services would *enable* her to stop driving? Toward that end I started calling around. Some central agency or organization must exist that would point me in the right direction to satisfy my mother's various driving needs. I imagined that, if not the government, then some or at least *one* of the big charities or organizations that are set up to help seniors could help my mother.

"You've been very sheltered," Rita told me with a fond and indulgent chuckle when I chronicled to her my dreary discoveries.

A, b, c...

"We don't offer that service. You might try X." "We don't offer that service. You might try Y." "You might try Z." "You might try Z-Minus-One." "You might try X."

"I've tried X."

"Oh. Have you tried A?"

"A? There's an ***A?****"*

"We don't offer that service. You might try B."

***

If Mother stopped driving, food would be her first priority. Meals on Wheels serves numerous people very well. But my mother had overcomc cancer and, she believed, kept it in remission partly by employing a particular, strict dietary regimen. This consisted of avoiding sugar, white flour and sundry processed foods; commencing every meal including breakfast with fresh, raw produce; and dinner salads with lettuce, broccoli, tomatoes, onions, carrots, celery, jicama, you name it: she'd come to love them all. But most of the Meals on Wheels cuisine was cooked, sugared, floured and/or otherwise processed. So Mother needed to shop for herself. Or else I needed to find an organization or individual who would either shop for her, following her instructions, or would take her shopping.

"And what about the specials?" Mother objected, obstructing my enterprise at its start. "How could I ask someone to pick up specials?" She discovered the specials she wanted by cruising down the supermarket aisles, and spontaneously scooped them up.

"Just tell whoever shops for you. 'Pick up any specials.'"

"But how would they know which one's I wanted?"

She wasn't going to make this easy.

But she did need to shop, get to the bank, her doctors and dentist, and to venture forth on whatever miscellaneous and unpredictable errands life presented. Who would help? Her car shot forward! The incident made me think again about contacting the Alzheimer's Association. They must have some volunteer service or at least know of one that would suit Mother's needs, even without a clinical diagnosis.

First, they sent me a list of support groups. But they were all too far for me to travel to and commenced too early in the morning for me to attend. As to my mother, she found it difficult enough to organize her time for what she considered essential. These groups never made the list.

The Alzheimer's Association also sent me a list of day care centers which would pick Mother up and keep her four to eight hours several days a week, the hours and days depending upon the center and the minimal money paid to it. But Mother spent her days reading, doing household chores, cooking—and her errands. She wasn't ready for a day care center even if it turned out she had Alzheimer's.

But no Alzheimer's Association list covered help with any of the driving services she needed.

Putting those lists aside, I started phoning Jewish groups, temples, churches, women's groups and government agencies. City, county, state, federal; but my mother lived too far east for help from one organization, too far north for another, or too far south and so on. One organization sent me a glossy brochure on how to donate money to them in one's will. The women's organization accorded no special services or assistance for elderly women in any region. Indeed, no central governmental or other organization or office I reached could provide a single, comprehensive list of organizations with services available to an elderly woman living alone in her particular district.

However, each call produced lists of possible organizations that might or might not assist Mother. Occasionally from within this haystack came the faint gleam of a potential needle of real help. I tracked down every one. Often, the organization or group at which I was aimed had nothing whatever to do with my mother's situation. But at last after some weeks, I unearthed two promising options, which I described to Mother.

"A local church has a driving program that can help, and the city has another. They're a little different, and they're both limited. It won't be like the independence you're used to. But between them you'll be okay."

"Well, that's very sweet of you, dear. It's something to keep in mind for the future."

"You need to think about it now," I advised yet again. In addition to her shaky mind, the cataracts in her eyes were getting worse. Driving at night, she saw a pale corona encircling everything.

"Very well," she replied with a deliberately literary phraseology. *Very well.* "I'll think about it."

"I don't know what to do," I told my friend, Camilla, a nurse practitioner I met through Suzann. I was terrified for Mother's possible crippling, pain and fear in the event of an accident, not to mention any possible victims. I mentioned Rita's suggestion of writing an anonymous letter to the DMV. "But I'd feel as if I'd betrayed her. And if she ever found out, she'd feel the same way."

Camilla recommended another possibility. "You could get her diagnosed by a doctor. By law, if a doctor believes a patient might be incompetent on the road, they have to notify the DMV."

I wondered if another foray into Mother's HMO would, this time, produce, instead of farce, a good doctor, one who could get Mother off the road and possibly even assist her with the mental disabilities she currently faced. This thought took root as mounting challenges stymied her.

Mounting Challenges

During the last decade my mother had acquired a series of hitches and glitches. Her osteoporosis exaggerated her scoliosis, put her on a cane, then a four-pronged cane, then a walker, and then bent her ever lower over her walker. In addition the shoulder injury from her upside down fall from the bar prevented her from reaching up with one arm, and her scoliosis thwarted her ability to lean over. The prosthesis in her left hip loosened further each day, making her walking increasingly painful and slow, and magnifying the chance of another fall. Her hearing had also diminished since her last bout of flu; the doctor decided to puncture her eardrums to release the fluid, and her eardrums never healed. And her memory gaps grew scarier yet.

For instance, Isela was Mother's friend, neighbor and "indispensable" household helper. "She keeps the house clean, the yard swept—and I don't know how else I'd ever get my groceries in." Using her walker, Mother could shop. But she'd finally given up trying to get her groceries into the house herself. Instead, at each store, bag upon bag amassed in her trunk, and there they would all remain until she could get into the house and call Isela, who would troop over with her six small children—"the mother and her little elves," as Mother described them. Isela removed Mother's cart from the trunk, piled the grocery bags into it and wheeled the lot to Mother's house.

The previous year Isela's family had to move from their nearby apartment. Mother told me, "Isela fought with her husband to move the family to a house within a block of me so she can keep helping me. Isn't that absolutely wonderful? What would I do without her?"

Now Mother said, "I never said that. She never did that!" If she could forget that, what else would she forget?

At my prompting she discovered where to obtain a free medic alert button to wear around her neck. She applied for one. "Press it," the issuers instructed her, "and someone will try to contact you by phone. If there's no answer, someone will go to your house immediately." However, there was a several-month waiting list for the free service, and Mother refused to pay thirty-five dollars for the private alert button. Until she got the free one, she had none.

My calls to her multiplied from twice a day to every couple of hours.

The Phone

I called in part to address the new loneliness in her that only I could assuage.

"You'll have to come over here and try this new dish I've made." "You'll have to come over here and see where I put the will and all the papers." "You'll have to come over here and see how the little wooden statuette on the table goes with the beautiful glass dish you gave me." "You'll have to come over and help me reorganize my shelves."

In the past, enjoying her deck with the birds, her reading and classical music, Mother could have lived without seeing another human soul for months. But now when one of her neighbors dropped by with a little dinner for her and a visit, she later shared the event with me in delight. But always it was me she wanted to see.

I did sometimes manage to get to her house when a friend drove me early in the day. I'd take the bus home. I used to bus over late in the day and Mitch, then Mother when Mitch was gone, would drive me home. But I no longer trusted Mother's driving; and at the same time, the incessant loud noise and virulent hostility toward me at my apartment had not abated, nor had my equally relentless insomnia. I couldn't drag myself out of bed early enough in the day to get to Mother's then get home on the bus before dark.

Justifying my continued absence, I described my newest upstairs neighbor.

"His crashing and banging went on for half an hour last night. I finally went up there. I had my little speech ready—'I'm sure you don't realize how the noise carries in this building,' blah, blah. *It was two thirty in the morning.* I knocked. Of course he knew it was me. Who else would it be? So instead of opening the door, he pounded back from his side—only once but so hard that the door panel popped toward me and then bounced back into the door. He broke the damn door! And the owners still won't say a word to him."

"Why do you suppose?"

"He pays his rent on time."

So did I, but my rent was a lot less because of Rent Control.

I'd looked for an apartment for month then gave up for the moment. But I was stuck in my skin as well as my apartment: a long-term sleep disorder is not about just being tired. I also tried to explain this to my mother. I had to make her understand. "Not sleeping day after day for years exhausts every cell and organ in your body. I have to rest up to go to the closet, rest up for the shower, rest up to put on what I've decided to wear, rest up to make food, rest up to eat it, rest up for the supplements afterwards." Sometimes I didn't get past resting up for the shower. "I eat and go back to bed." My thighs were too weak to keep the rest of me going. On the days I felt a little stronger, I remained concerned about pushing myself into cancer or a heart attack with my underlying virus. Instead of visiting, I called my mother constantly and, when not justifying my absence, I visited with her on the phone.

I asked how she was, asked her advice on such-and-such, gave her my own advice, called to share a joke. I called to pass on news I'd heard on the radio she might not have heard or to tell her what interesting program was on. I also shared with Mother my latest writing ventures, to each of which she responded the same way. "That's nice, dear. I certainly wish you luck." I smiled. I'd have preferred the ecstatic "Oh!" my jewelry elicited. But this blank check of mindless maternal good will did not offend or anger me. That was how I realized how much *I'd* changed.

In the process of each call, I made sure she was okay.

I called to make sure she hadn't fallen down and wasn't lying somewhere unable to rise or reach the phone. I called to make sure she hadn't forgotten she'd left the stove on and burned down the house. I called to make sure some other catastrophe hadn't hurtled her into diverse unforeseen perils.

I was always anxious. Anything might happen.

My fears for her especially surfaced during power blackouts. When the power went out anywhere in Los Angeles, it invariably hit her neighborhood first. I imagined her tripping in the dark and falling or, worse yet, dropping one of the candles she insisted on lighting during blackouts even though she was deathly afraid of fire. On the walker now, she'd never be able to move fast enough either to put out or flee a fire.

"Just use flashlights!" Of course, my words rebounded uselessly against the wall of her amiable intransigence.

"Oh, I'll be all right. It'll be fine, dear. Don't worry."

Oh, okay. That makes me feel so much better.

She left her phone off the hook and didn't notice for hours; went to her desk or outside to the deck or into the service porch and forgot to bring the cordless with her; or she had the cordless, but it didn't ring. The call shuttled directly to the answering machine, which she couldn't hear and wouldn't check for hours. Sometimes the answering machine failed to pick up.

Her phone had various disabilities of its own. Static might rage as we talked. Or the connection died altogether. When I called, her line often rang busy when it shouldn't, since she had Call Waiting. Each of these events prompted me to call the phone company.

They informed me, "We can't tell if the phone isn't working or it's off the hook." They instructed me, "When this happens she needs to disconnect the cord at the phone and also at the jack, wait five minutes, then reconnect it. If that doesn't work, call us back."

I told them, "My mother has four phones, one in every room, she's disabled, she can't reach any of the jacks, and she wouldn't be able to retain all these instructions anyway. I'll see if I can find a neighbor to send over to her, but meanwhile let me make an appointment for you to go to her house. If her neighbor fixes the phone, I'll call you back and cancel the appointment."

If no neighbor was home or it was too late to bother them, I called the police. "Could you please go to my mother's house and check on her?" I asked them also to please pass on to Mother the appointment date I'd made for her with the phone company.

The phone company replaced by mail one after another of Mother's disabled phones, but they never sent anyone to pick up their disabled phones for the disabled. Susie and I, in our Saturday sorting and digging, already have found three of them in Mother's closet.

By the time my mother got her medic alert system six months before her operation, my calling her constantly had become an unbreakable habit to give her emotional support if nothing else, since I couldn't give it in person.

***

Forget the hazards of her falling. The simple dysfunctions of her daily life broke my heart when she told me about them. If she dropped a file folder, she had to use her reacher, a long gadget with pincers at the end, to pick up every single piece of paper. If she dropped a plate of food, she had only her reacher to pick up the chunks, and her feet to move the rag around the floor. "My mouth was just *watering* for that chicken!" She was practically in tears. "Now it'll take me hours just to clean up the mess!"

"Just to put on my shoes," she explained, "I have to lie on my back on the bed, pull my feet up and tug my shoes over my feet. At least I don't have shoelaces. This is a terrible way to live!" she said with a little laugh, but meant it.

I suggested, "Why don't you consider clearing out the small, spare bedroom so someone can live with you?"

Her response each time I submitted this idea was predictable. She laughed. I didn't. There was only one aspect of my suggestion upon which we agreed.

"People are always asking me why you can't come live with me. What a disaster that would be!"

Mother's friends queried me in the same way. None of them understood why *I* couldn't live with her and help her. How I longed to do just that! But Mother's house was packed to the square nano-inch, and she had no clue what to get rid of to make room for me. Nor had she any desire whatever to get rid of anything, while at the same time I had my own apple-from-the-same-tree heaps and throngs of *things.* What would I leave behind? On top of which neither of us could imagine living in such close quarters with each other when we both valued our privacy and were so set in our ways.

And of course there always remained the transportation problem of living in Echo Park. How would I get anywhere in any remotely reasonable period of time; the very problem Mother would face if she quit driving and that I would face today should I keep the house? So I did what guilt and love compelled me to do. Unaware of the gargantuan magnitude of my recommendation, I offered, "If you let someone move into the little bedroom, I'll help you clear it out." Then, with a quick if unusual instinct, I added, "We'll bring in Isela. We'll pay her to help us."

However, as unwaveringly as Mother rejected giving up her car, she refused any notion of anyone moving in. "I couldn't live with anyone! My privacy is everything! There isn't room! What would I say to them? And I don't want to spend money on that! Do you know how much we have left?"

"No."

"Not enough. How much would it cost?"

"A lot," I had to admit.

"Well, when the time comes that I need someone, we'll talk about it."

"This is the time."

"I love you for your concern and I do appreciate it. But. No. It's not."

I called the local church I'd discovered that had the driving program that Mother refused to consider. Elsa, the geriatric social worker there, recommended a "senior companion." I related to Mother Elsa's definition. "A senior companion is someone who volunteers to keep the elderly company. The church can send someone at no cost. She would come visit you a few hours a day. If you fell or hurt yourself, she could call the fire department or whoever." If Mother got used to that, I added silently, maybe she would think about live-in help.

"Will they help me with the dishes or cooking?"

"No. They're not permitted to do actual work."

"Then they would just make my life harder. I'd have to *make conversation.*" This, from the woman who spent hours daily talking on the phone when she wasn't searching for a missing item—which a senior companion could help her find.

"No, you wouldn't," I asserted, remembering Dorothy. When I was a child, Dorothy was one of the series of women Mother had hired to take care of me while she worked and went to night school. Dorothy was intelligent, kind, politically sympatico with Mother, and she read the same things my mother found interesting. Also, Dorothy respected other people's space. Someone like her would never impose. "I never know if I'm doing the right thing," Dorothy once told me, "so I don't feel qualified to tell anyone else what to do." Dorothy became Mother's and my lifetime friend.

"I'll find someone who enjoys reading. A woman who can just sit with you on the porch and read while you read. If you drop a plate or file or something, she could retrieve it for you."

"No, no. Someone else would just get in the way."

"I'll search until I find someone like Dorothy."

"I don't need someone to *sit with me,"* Mother cut me off with insulted vehemence.

But of course she did. "You know," I explored tentatively, "there's another possibility. If you sold the house, we could take an apartment together in the Fairfax area. I could help you, and you'd have all your shopping in walking distance. Food stores, book stores, and there are all kinds of Jewish senior centers and activities." As I spoke, this prospect took on an idyllic character in my mind, a veritable aurora bathing me in joy just contemplating the advantages Mother would gain, and how wonderful it would be to be able to help her. We could share a two-bedroom; and Fairfax was a neighborhood with do-able bus routes.

"I'd rather die than move."

The paradise I envisioned began dwindling toward the sweet and distant Shangri La of one of our favorite movies, *Lost Horizons*.

Meanwhile, at Elsa's suggestion I ordered an identification bracelet for Mother from a free service. For the incidents of dementia, rare up to this point, began to worsen; and although it seemed impossible, I had to concede that at least theoretically Elsa was right when she said, "She might wander off and forget who she is."

Renewed Quest

I also resumed my search for a doctor who'd give Mother the correct diagnosis. We needed to know what we were dealing with. While I lacked faith in orthodox medical treatments, I did value their testing. If we could discover what specific condition or disease was causing her symptoms, we could research what holistic medicines might help. (That is, she could research, and I would encourage her.)

A doctor who specialized in the elderly might also persuade her to try a senior companion; give her a few behavior modification techniques to deal with her stress, especially the frenzy that compelled her hours-long searches for misplaced items; and convince her to stop driving or, failing that, notify the DMV. Finally, I pictured this imaginary doctor helping Mother deal with the trauma of facing her mental condition, should it prove permanent.

These rosy doctor scenarios, however, entailed a different doctor than the one she saw the previous year, when Mother had surprised me with her receptiveness to the idea of getting a diagnosis.

***

"No one's said I have Alzheimer's," she kept telling me at the time; I knew she was afraid. If a doctor did tell her she had it, she could no longer deny it. When I suggested to her that she make an appointment with a gerontologist, I expected her to balk. But she knew something was seriously amiss, she couldn't stand forgetting things all the time, and she too wanted to know what was wrong.

Or perhaps that's putting it too strongly. What she actually said was, "Well, it wouldn't hurt to find out." So I'd called Dr. Burns, the oncologist who was her regular doctor at her HMO. Burns had saved my mother's life at least once. After a bowel obstruction operation a few years before, the hospital doctor in charge of Mother checked the mechanical and electronic monitors. These indicated, as Mother lay in the hospital panting with each and every breath, that she was doing okay. He never physically examined my mother. Dr. Burns did, however. Visiting Mother daily, she discovered that Mother was losing too much fluid and corrected the situation before it killed her.

So now I phoned Dr. Burns and described the memory problems I was seeing in Mother, which at that time consisted mostly of forgotten words, vanished items and her obsessive searches. I asked Burns if she could give my mother a referral to a specialist. The doctor agreed to do so.

A few weeks later, returning home from her appointment with the gerontologist Burns had arranged for her to see, Mother called me and related to my optimistic ears her HMO adventure. "He didn't know why I was there."

My optimistic ears drooped. "It wasn't in your file?"

"Apparently not." (When I told Burns about this, her anger was palpable. "All he had to do was pick up a phone and call me.") "I told him I wasn't sure why I was there, either," Mother said. "I said I guessed my daughter was worried about Alzheimer's. He asked me a few questions. When he found out I read a lot, he told me, 'Oh, if you read, you don't have Alzheimer's.'"

I crossed my eyes. A surfeit of possibilities, in which a person with Alzheimer's still reads, sprinted through my mind.

"Then later on in the interview," Mother continued, "I commented that something or other was 'palliative.' The doctor laughed. He said, 'If you use words like *palliative,* you don't have Alzheimer's.' He told me not to worry. He said I could tell you I'm okay."

I thought, *What an idiot.*

Mother sounded relieved as she related this medical assessment, but at the same time she gave a sarcastic laugh. Whatever was wrong with her brain, her cognitive functions remained sufficiently intact to analyze the doctor's own mental shortcoming and to convey her thinking, which came across lucidly: *What an idiot.*

"I told him," she further recounted, "that I'm always misplacing things and I spend hours looking for them. Sometimes they completely disappear."

"Did you tell him you make yourself a frantic total wreck looking for them? How you don't eat or stop even when your blood is pounding in your ears?"

"Well... I don't think so. I don't remember," she confessed sheepishly.

"What did he say about the misplaced items?"

"He said, 'People who have Alzheimer's think other people have moved them, and they call the police.' 'Oh, no,' I told him in disgust, 'I know who's doing it. It's me.'" She sounded more willing to accept his medical reassurances in these circumstances. So was I: Finally, a facet of the examination made sense.

At the end of her interview the doctor diagnosed her with Parkinson's-like Syndrome, which means exactly what it sounds like. It's not clinically Parkinson's. But it exhibits most or all of the symptoms of Parkinson's. Since the doctors don't know what the problem actually is, that's what they call it. Parkinson's-like Syndrome.

The doctor gave her a prescription for it. Once home, however, Mother looked up the side effects of the prescribed drug in her PDR. The Physician's Desk Reference lists numerous drugs, their uses, contra-indications, side effects and so on. She always looked everything up. She found that the potential side effects included the blurred vision and dizziness that appears at the beginning of so many printouts of side effects on so many other drugs and that could prove fatal for an old woman living alone should she become dizzy and fall. And of course: "Don't drive if you have any of these symptoms," the instructions read. "I'll get by without it," she resolved of the drug, expressing no conflict in her decision.

Well, she'd said of seeing a doctor, *it wouldn't hurt.* It didn't. *That,* I'd thought, *is about the best one can say.*

During the next year her driving problems had worsened, culminating in the unexplained acceleration in her HMO garage. Then, more recently, her memory further stagnated. During one of our telephone conversations, I mentioned something about her lymphoma.

"Oh, is that what I had? Oh, isn't that interesting! I never knew that!"

But she was the one who told me.

I kept silent. Why torment her by pointing out such a crucial forgetting?

Then came the quantum jump toward the void. "I was just sitting here! I just had that paper in my hand! I haven't moved from the table and it is just nowhere. *No! Where!"*

"Are you sure?"

"Of course I'm sure."

"And you haven't left the table."

"No!" she insisted, irate and frustrated.

"Well, a poltergeist didn't move it," I reminded her, expecting laughter. She often joked about how "a poltergeist" must live with her, moving her things around.

She responded in all seriousness, "Well... I don't know."

My head was spinning. "It wasn't a poltergeist."

She was silent.

I felt as if someone had pulled a plug and solid reality had suddenly liquified and was swirling away down the drain. Then there occurred the first event which brought to mind the idiot gerontologist. His one decent bit of information about Alzheimer's came back to me as if it had been a prophecy. Mother started calling the police.

Mild Dementia

"When I came home from the store, someone had gone through all the drawers in my bedroom! I'm shaking so badly I can hardly talk. The drawers of my chest, the brown chest, they were all open, and everything was a mess. Someone tossed my clothes all over the bed and floor. And there on my bed sat my little carrying case!"

It was the same carrying case she had discovered in the closet a few weeks before. She'd remarked to me, "I forgot all about this! Next time I have to go to the hospital I can use it."

As she described the "break-in," I thought, *She was looking for something in a frenzy, found the case, then went to the store and forgot the whole episode.*

"I waited a few hours until I calmed down," she went on. "Then I called the police."

The police. "What did they say?"

"What could they say? They wrote it up."

A month later Mother woke up in the night to see someone in a long white gown standing in the doorway to her bedroom. The figure turned and fled. "Whoever it was left the minute I saw them. I just saw the white like an afterimage as the person raced away."

"What did you do?" Fear for her mind made me queasy. But at the same time, so did the faint possibility that an intruder had really been there and endangered my mother's life.

But her own entire terror focused on the menace she'd faced from the supposed invader. "I got up and went into the living room. I was wobbly with terror. Whoever was there was gone. But the front door was unlocked. And there on the kitchen table," she proclaimed in undiminished dread but with equal indignation, "in total disarray, were all my bills and checks, all mixed up. Can you imagine the nerve of someone!" she demanded. "They just come in and sit down at my table and mix up all my checks and bills!"

My fear for her life, posed by a possible intruder, vanished, replaced by the desire to cry. "Why would a stranger do that?" How could she fail to see her own irrationality? How could she leave me alone with this anguished comprehension of what was going on?

"How should I know!" she snapped. "Just to drive me crazy!"

And paranoid as well.

My voice gentle, I broached the possibility that perhaps she'd done it herself. "Maybe you were working on the checks, got tired and went to bed. And forgot."

She rejected the notion immediately. "Then who was in the doorway?"

"Maybe you were dreaming." I didn't say hallucinating. "Maybe you were still half in a dream when you woke up."

"Then who turned on the lamp? The lamp by the bedroom door was on when I woke up!"

"Maybe you went to the bathroom and back to bed without turning the lamp off, and the light is what woke you."

She began to withdraw. "Well, if you don't care what happens to me..."

"Of course I care! I'm just not sure..."

"Never mind. I'm sorry I told you." Abandonment and betrayal dulled her voice.

"I'm sorry. I have to tell you what I think."

"Of course you do."

But did I? Over the next days, the more I tried to get her to consider the possibility that she "dreamed" the white-gowned intruder, and that she had moved the checks and bills around herself and forgotten, the more hurt she felt, the more abandoned and unloved. I didn't know what to do. I called Elsa, the church geriatric social worker, to ask her if *she* would try to convince Mother to face what was happening to her. But on the day Elsa came to Mother's house to meet her, I happened to be visiting Mother. She had misplaced something else, which she thought someone might have come in and taken. "Well," suggested Elsa, "let's just look around and see if we can find it."

Anger tightened my muscles. Why didn't Elsa try to make Mother see she had done it herself? Mother needed to start dealing with her symptoms. And I needed Elsa's help getting Mother to do this. Of course they couldn't find whatever Mother had lost, and she was distraught.

On other visits about which I heard from my mother on the phone, Elsa continued to avoid confronting Mother's irrationality head-on. I was shocked. How could my mother deal with reality if everyone supported her denial of it?

Or was Elsa right? Maybe this *was* the way to handle a person with her condition. Whenever I expressed to Mother my fear she might have some dementia, the only result of my directness was her further emotional withdrawal. "I'd be relieved to think it was me!" she professed of each new event. "I'm terrified! But why would I do that?"

"You might have Alzheimer's." I spoke with intense focus, as if by the forceful pronunciation of my words I could chisel their meaning into her mind. "It's a symptom of Alzheimer's—doing irrational things and then forgetting. So how would you remember strange things you've done if a disease makes you forget them?"

But my reasoning wounded her ever more deeply. "You think I'm crazy!" "Well, if you don't care what happens to me..." "If you don't care if I die..."

Moreover, I was still not absolutely, totally certain she'd hallucinated *all* of it.

Calling the Police

Suppose Mother was right? Suzann told me, "Sometimes thieves and vandals do weird things when they break in. You'd be surprised." And there'd been genuine thefts. A box Mother couldn't have lifted had been removed from the porch. A large pot she couldn't have dislodged had been stolen from the yard. What if someone *was* out there? What if she was in danger?

I told her one night, "The next time something happens, call the police immediately. Don't wait. Let them decide professionally what's going on."

The next morning Mother awoke to discover, "Someone broke in and went through my purse! They stole the thirty dollars that was in there! They took my purse from my bedroom." She was shaking, sick and weak with terror. "They took my purse into the living room and emptied it. Everything was all over the floor! And my money is gone! They stole my money! If I'd woken while they were there—if I'd seen who it was and they knew it—I don't even want to think about what they would have done to me." She had immediately called the police.

A well of desolation opened inside me. The timing was just too suspicious. I tell her, "Next time call the police immediately." And that very night, *hours later,* there's another incident which justifies her calling the police, to prove her point. It was someone else. It wasn't her.

My helplessness grew with the avalanche of incidents. "My checkbook is gone!" Her voice on the phone, high with hysteria, filled with tears. "Someone came in here last night and stole my checkbook!" She called the police again. On their advice she changed the locks on the door, terminated that checking account and started another one.

Then she misplaced the spares of her new keys. A few weeks later they turned up mysteriously. "When I came home, a whole slew of keys were lined up neatly on the deck table. The ones I just had made and couldn't find—and a whole bunch of rusty, old keys I've never seen before in my life! The chair was pulled out for someone to sit down there. Can you imagine?" Fear and indignation vied once more for prominence. "Someone just sat down and made themselves at home and lined up these keys!"

"But..." My attempt to engage her in a rational discussion was becoming as compulsive and irrational as hers to prove her sanity. But I was desperate. Somehow I felt if I could make her reason out her dementia, I would pull her back to me. "You won't want to hear this. But maybe you did it and don't remember."

"I would remember," she countered scornfully. "Anyway, I've never seen those old keys before in my life. Where would I get them?"

"You could have found them in a drawer or closet or the service porch." I was becoming angry at her unwillingness to be logical. "I have no idea."

"But why would I leave them out there like that?" she cross-examined, in the style of communication she learned during her decades typing transcriptions of civil lawsuits. "What possible reason could I have for doing that?"

"With Alzheimer's you wouldn't *have* a reason."

"I'll show you the keys, and *you* tell me where they came from! *Just look at them and tell me where I could have gotten them.*"

"It doesn't matter what they look like!!!"

I described the event to my friend, Maya, whose aunt had had Alzheimer's. She confirmed my feeling about these keys as well as the carrying case of a few weeks before. "That's just what would happen to my aunt. Your mother probably became fixated on the keys for some reason, messed around with them, left them and forgot all about it. My aunt was always doing stuff like that."

The next month Mother discovered her "stolen" checkbook at the back of a drawer in her bedroom vanity. She had no memory of putting it there, let alone any idea why she'd done it. The quiet defeat in her voice, when she admitted finding it, told me she knew she was sliding farther down the slick, bleak slope.

I encouraged her to see another doctor. "Let me arrange it. Let's get a decent diagnosis this time." Tactfully I refrained from bringing up the painful issue of her possible dementia. "If we know why you're having these memory problems, we can research some holistic method for treating it."

I didn't tell her what I'd learned by this time from Camilla, the nurse practitioner: A doctor who found my mother mentally incompetent was legally obligated to report her to the DMV. If holistic medicine failed to reverse whatever was happening to her mind, I wanted, at the least, someone other than me to get her out from behind the wheel.

Dr. Burns

I related to Dr. Burns Mother's current measure of forgetfulness. "It's like the Twilight Zone," I said. "Whole segments of her memory are disappearing from her mind like sand castles washed away at the edge of the sea."

Burns communicated to me a few similar incidents she'd seen herself when Mother came for a check-up.

I said, "It's not just her memory, either." I hesitated. After the incident with the keys, the whole subject of Mother's dementia had become so painful and sensitive, so dangerous to our relationship, that it threatened to tear us apart. I'd stopped trying to reason with my mother and avoided thinking about it as much as possible. However, I now had no choice.

"She's had a few of what seem to me—hallucinations." I related those incidents. "I don't know what to do, how to talk to her. I'm just floundering. She needs professional help to deal with it. We both need to talk to a specialist. But not that doctor she saw last time." I didn't say, *That idiot.* But, apparently, Dr. Burns remembered.

"I'll set up an appointment for another gerontologist. In fact, I'll arrange for your mother to have the three-hour, in-depth gerontology exam."

On the big day Mother and I spent most of the three hours waiting for the HMO specialist.

The In-Depth Exam

When I joined Mother in the exam room ten minutes late, I found her sitting on the exam table in her hospital gown, exhausted from the stress of making herself do the impossible: arrive anywhere on time. We chatted for half an hour before the doctor's assistant arrived.

A pleasant, dark-haired woman in her late twenties, she informed us, "I'm going to take the initial notes. Then I'll talk to the doctor. Then he'll come in to see you."

So Mother described how she lost names, words and things. But she said nothing about the big-ticket items, the mysterious keys, the "stolen" checkbook, the white-gowned intruder, the car leaping forward.

Quietly, so that Mother couldn't hear, I added, "And things happen that in my opinion might be dementia."

The assistant wrote down everything we said, asking no questions. I decided to volunteer nothing further. I'd wait and discuss the full picture with the gerontologist himself. There was finally going to be someone with answers. He would be able to tell me how I should deal with Mother's symptoms as they arose, without triggering her anger and withdrawal. He'd be able to describe what further symptoms might appear, at what rate, and so on; and how I could help.

The assistant left.

Mother and I waited and chatted, chatted and waited. "This is taking forever," I complained.

"It certainly is."

When the doctor finally entered the room, he introduced himself and got right to work.

***

While he popped the blood pressure unit onto Mother's arm, he declared, "We'll go over everything when

I've finished my exam." Taking her blood pressure, he listened as Mother repeated her story about losing names and words and misplacing objects. From his non-response, it was unclear to Mother and me whether the assistant had informed him of the symptoms we'd described to her. I said, "And she gets so stressed about it." More tenuously, and quietly, I added, "And there are things that—scare me."

"Go ahead," the doctor stated, examining my mother briskly, holding her wrists, tapping her knees, telling her to move her eyes this way or her hands that way. Moving right along. His back to me. "I'm listening."

I faltered. Any more explicit words than those I'd just spoken, about being scared, any further detail about my mother's dementia, would again touch her raw nerve. It was the weakest link in our relationship. I needed the doctor's full attention so we could *talk.* I thought, *I'll wait until he's done and we all sit on the other side of his desk and "go over everything."*

He finished the physical exam, which took about fifteen minutes, to give him the benefit of the doubt. "I don't see any signs of Parkinson's-like Syndrome," he declared, unconditionally contradicting the first gerontologist. Then he gave Mother a piece of paper and pencil. He instructed her, "Can you draw a clock with the hands at 2:30?"

Hesitantly, she drew a handless clock. Pausing, she fiddled with the pencil, frowning in concentration. I stared at her, dumbstruck at seeing her struggle so hard with this simple task. Finally, she filled in the numbers and hands correctly.

The doctor checked the paper then asked, "Can you name the President of the United States?"

At this, she spoke correctly and without hesitation.

The doctor left for another large block of time. Mother and I chatted and waited. When the doctor returned, he told my mother, "Come back in six months."

There was no "other side of his desk" in his office. This was it. The summing up. The discussion of "everything." The "in-depth" interview. Bye-bye.

Our waiting must have constituted the epoch it seemed because despite the brevity of the doctor's examination, when Mother and I eventually left the clinic, her watch told us that three hours had passed since we'd arrived.

I called Dr. Burns the next day and relayed the events. She promised to arrange for Mother to see a neurologist. Before that visit came about, I encountered Ruthie at the Monday farmers' market. We hadn't seen each other for several weeks. We traded the latest news. Ruthie told me her mother's Alzheimer's had entered the late stage. "She can't wear plaid or flowers or any pattern or bright color because she becomes fixated on it. She becomes obsessed with trying to scratch it off her clothes."

"I'm so sorry," I told her. At the same time, anger flared up in me for Mother's sake. This was exactly the kind of specific behavior I needed to know, that I'd sought in vain from Mother's doctors and the Alzheimer's Association. How did that fixation look early on? Was my mother's insatiable obsession to find misplaced articles an example of it and if so, how could I help her? Why was it so hard to get basic information?

Then there transpired the episode of dementia that conspicuously unnerved Mother and in fact must have terrified her in her secret, deepest interstices. This was the one she was helpless to deny.

The Note

Her research into holistic and conventional medicine for the brain unearthed data about a pharmaceutical called Aricept. "There are a lot of studies on it." Her excitement crackled over the phone. "They're using it in England to treat age-related memory loss and Alzheimer's. It looks so promising! I want to try it, but Dr. Burns won't give it to me."

"Why not?"

"She says it's dangerous. But she never says why. She never has time to discuss it. I want to try it!" She continued to pester Dr. Burns for a prescription then decided to get the information herself. She went to her HMO pharmacy and asked for a printout on the drug. After reading it she decided, "You know what? Dr. Burns is right."

At the top of the list of possible side effects came once more the notorious blurred vision and dizziness. "That's all I'd need," Mother said dryly, rejecting it as she had done the drug prescribed by the first gerontologist, for "Parkinson's-like Syndrome."

The next time Mother saw Dr. Burns, she handed her the computer printout. "You're right. I'm not going to take this!"

A few days later, Mother was getting something out of her purse and found the printout. Scribbled at the bottom was a note. "I want to take this drug for my Parkinson's-like Syndrome." The note sent a chill down to her toes. It made no sense. Mother had obtained the printout on Aricept *after* she'd learned from the "in-depth" interview that she didn't have Parkinson's-like Syndrome. Then, upon reading the printout, she'd decided against taking the drug. Most eerily, however, the handwriting wasn't hers. "And the first letter of some of the words is capitalized. I'd never do that!"

No, with her meticulous and indisputable level of literacy, she never would. "I know." *Never.* Yet she had to have done it.

She continued to deny she had Alzheimer's or any form of dementia.

"But how did that writing get on that paper if you didn't put it there?"

"I don't know."

"This is *really weird.*"

"I couldn't agree more."

I heard the fear and confusion in her voice. She couldn't conceive that she might have written the note. But simultaneously she knew it couldn't have been anyone else.

"This is the most frightening thing yet," I said.

"Yes, it is." Her agreement was subdued. The note forced her to concede, if only temporarily, the frightful weirdness of the whole glut of recent events.

The day came for her appointment with the new neurologist to whom Burns was sending her. This new doctor diagnosed Mother with early Alzheimer's and prescribed Aricept. After a week Mother said she would take it after all. "I have to do something." She admitted then that she was already taking it at night. "If I have a problem, it won't affect my driving."

"What about going to the bathroom all night and maybe falling?"

A pause. "Well. It hasn't happened." She didn't care. She wanted her mind back and would take any risk.

The Diagnostician

One morning last month I heard a radio interview featuring Jacqueline Marcell, author of *Elder Rage, or Take My Father…Please!* She offered a great deal of information about elder care, but what struck me most was her experience with the Alzheimer's Association. They had informed her about medications that slow the progression of Alzheimer's Disease: Aricept, Exelon, Razadyne and Namenda. Jacqueline said that once her father's brain chemistry was properly balanced and slowing the dementia, and his depression and aggression were also medically treated, he was much easier to manage. I listened in amazement, grief and anger because in all the calls I'd made to the Association, they never volunteered this information; and it had never occurred to me to ask about medications other than Aricept that might help my mother, that she might at least want to investigate.

However, the Alzheimer's Association did send me, along with their lists of day care centers, a little pamphlet. It said that, at best, you could only confirm an Alzheimer's diagnosis with eighty to ninety percent precision. Only after death, from an autopsy, could the presence of Alzheimer's be proven incontestably. Moreover, to achieve that eighty to ninety percent accuracy, the patient requires a CT-scan, an MRI and a team psychiatric evaluation.

Mother's new neurologist, the only doctor to make the Alzheimer's determination, gave her only one long written test during her one and only visit, and a CT-scan. Yet she unequivocally diagnosed Mother with Alzheimer's.

As a character in a Robert Barnard mystery novel declares, "Well, it's an opinion, I suppose."

Attempting to get it substantiated, I left four calls for the neurologist, requesting she give Mother an MRI and team psychiatric exam. I still believed that with the right information, Mother had a chance to turn her symptoms around. I also expected that if Mother did have Alzheimer's, then *this* doctor could tell me what to look for in the progress of the disease and what to do at its various stages. You know. We could consult.

Last month, seeking to understand what happened to Mother, I acquired documents from her HMO. I saw that the neurologist noted in my mother's chart that she intended to contact "the daughter," me, and discuss her findings. But she'd never returned my calls, let alone initiated one. And—not even to protect herself—she made no mention of Mother's driving.

The neurologist had a patient, my mother, whom she'd diagnosed with "mild" Alzheimer's. One symptom of Alzheimer's is impaired judgment. My mother was extremely conscientious her whole life. In her right mind she would have recognized herself as a hazard to others on the road. She'd never have continued driving. But by definition, Alzheimer's precludes judgment. Both legally and morally, the doctor was responsible for doing what my mother couldn't. Yet she'd made no effort whatsoever to notify the DMV.

Apparently it's common practice for physicians to leave this unpleasant duty to the family, indeed, in some cases, to dump it there in the most unconscionable manner.

But I would learn only with the next doctor that when dealing with an elderly loved one who must stop driving, you must be absolutely sure of the professional you're dealing with before you open your mouth about it. Take a hint. If the doctor shows no inclination to notify the DMV without your urging, you can probably take it as the salient sign of a pattern, one that may eventually erupt in emotional upheaval.

The Psychiatrist

My conscience demanded I anonymously notify the DMV about Mother. They would probably seize her license and save lives. But the more her mind broke down, the more helpless she felt, and the more my anxiety grew at the consequences of such a step should she ever find out. She'd feel more alone and vulnerable than she did when I expressed doubt that "someone broke into" her house. She'd never overcome her feeling of being betrayed by the person she loved most. Before I risked that, I decided to make one last effort in my quest for a physician's help.

Calling the psychology department at Mother's HMO, by chance I reached the department head. I told her about my mother, outlined the questions I had about Alzheimer's, and presented my need for someone other than me to get Mother off the road. The woman running the department said, "We have a psychiatrist who specializes in geriatric psychiatry. I think Dr. Stevens is just the right person."

An airy, joyous relief breezed through me. What better type of doctor, I thought, to help Mother come to terms with her failing memory and the episodes of dementia? Who better to help her find ways to cope with her new reality—including accepting someone to live with her—at least until she found a way to eliminate her Alzheimer's symptoms? Moreover, a geriatric psychiatrist would have *resources.* She could offer alternatives to Mother's driving that I'd been unable to find. When Stevens felt my mother was ready to give up her car, *she* would notify the DMV.

Dream on.

Mother went for her first appointment with Stevens. She called me about it that night. "What did you talk about?" I asked eagerly.

"I don't know," said my mother. "She asked me some questions."

"About what?"

"I guess about how I forget things... I don't remember." She laughed.

That was it.

The next day I left a message for Stevens. "My mother needs to stop driving, and this can't come from me. This is urgent. Please call me!" I left the message three times. When she called, I would discuss the other issues. Perhaps we could work out a plan together. When she didn't return any of my calls, I joined my mother for her second visit.

A Trip to the Psychiatrist

Appearing in the waiting room at the assigned time, I found Mother had not yet arrived. By now she was *never* on time for *anything*. I decided to take advantage of her tardiness, asking the receptionist if I could see Dr. Stevens for a minute.

Behind the receptionist, on her side of the window, an attractive young woman in her mid-thirties glanced over at me, seeming to respond to the name "Dr. Stevens." Then she turned and left the receptionist's cubicle, diminishing into the farther recesses of the many offices and exam rooms. The receptionist went after her. Returning, she explained, "Dr. Stevens can't talk to you about your mother until she gets your mother's written consent."

"Okay." I thought, *Good start*. Then, "Can she just give me some general information on Alzheimer's and general care instructions, like that?"

"You'll have to wait for your mother."

"But it's just general information."

"You'll have to wait."

I took a seat in the waiting room, the well of hope in my heart already starting to evaporate. Mother arrived an hour later, highly stressed because she was so late. Her stress detonated when she opened her purse to extract her co-payment. It was missing. "I had twenty dollars! I put a twenty in here last night!" Her voice cracked as she verged on tears. She was ready to cry from frustration at having to get there on time, compounded by fresh fear for her mind, or for some new "theft."

"It's all right," I told her, a hand on her fragile shoulder. "You can mail it in."

"But I put it in here last night."

"It's all right." I kissed her soft cheek.

Stevens, who indeed turned out to be the woman I'd seen earlier, came out to the waiting room and invited us back into her office. She sat Mother on one side of the room and me on the other. She spoke in a normal volume but had turned her back to Mother, who was leaning forward and kept saying, "I can't hear you. What are you saying? I can't hear you."

I looked at Mother and back to Stevens. This physical arrangement seemed not only stupid but cruel. "She can't hear us." I couldn't suppress my anger. "I thought the whole point of your not talking to me first was that you needed my mother's permission. Now you're ignoring her."

At this challenge to her authority, Stevens transformed. Her shoulders stiffened. Her eyelids fluttered furiously. I could almost see her sparking, smoking, jerking and generally shorting out like a *Star Trek* android. Once she got herself back under control, she spoke with a canned professionalism, a patronizing smile. "Let's just proceed. I'm here to help you."

She sounded so normal, in her own way, that I doubted myself. I knew my nerves were raw. Maybe I was being unfair, judging her too soon and too much by previous doctors. "Okay. My mother is really upset right now." If she could help, I wanted to give her every opportunity. "She mislaid the money she was going to bring here today for co-payment, and she's really upset about it."

Stevens turned to my mother. They spoke briefly. I no longer recall what they said. First, I was dumbfounded by Stevens' inadequacy. She made no attempt to lead Mother into an in-depth discussion about her symptoms when this was the perfect opportunity. Second, what came next was so traumatic that it knocked their minor conversation out of my mind for all time.

Stevens turned back to me and remarked, at normal volume, "I understand you're concerned about your mother's driving. You don't think she should drive."

Panic drained the blood from my face. *My mother was right there. She could hear this!*

"You want my help to stop her from driving," Stevens went on.

Had I been standing, I'd have passed out from the dizziness overwhelming me. How could she say that in front of Mother after all the messages I'd left her? How could she endanger my relationship with my mother like this? She was a psychiatrist. She was supposed to be sensitive to people's emotions. She was supposed have some clue to people's thinking. To their, oh, *psychology.*

I glanced at my mother from the corner of my eye. She continued leaning forward in the corner chair where Stevens had stationed her. Her face was constricted with tension, anger and a growing dejection as she strained and failed to hear us.

An ache throbbed in my throat. Mother looked so helpless and miserable… But I might escape this disaster.

And here is where my own lunacy prevailed, some version of which would persist throughout Mother's whole hellish journey because although my mother and I had become two different people in our relationship, a part of my psyche remained untouched by any change. I never learned what my mother had learned: to trust my instincts.

My Lunacy

Rather than marching Mother out of Stevens's office right then and there, I did what this Doctor, as the Authority Figure of All Authority Figures, expected. I behaved as if Stevens deserved my trust. In my quietest voice, casting fleeting glances at Mother to make sure she couldn't hear me, I outlined the dangers I felt she posed as a driver.

As Stevens and I spoke, Stevens kept her back to Mother, whose frustration at being unable to hear, and whose anger and humiliation at being ignored, drove her once more to the edge of tears. Meeting disrespect had become her common experience of being an old woman in our culture, and she hated it.

When I finished the litany of the events that concerned me, Stevens turned to Mother. "We're a little concerned about your driving. I'd like to send a form to the DMV." She handed the form to my mother and asked her to sign it.

Mother took it tentatively. She'd missed the "we."

"They'll probably want to interview you. Do you understand? Is that all right?"

Mother nodded vaguely, her expression wary. At least she was now included in the conversation. "I guess so." She took the paper. In her whole life she'd never signed anything without reading it thoroughly. But this time, resentful, confused and trusting me, and perhaps intimidated just a little by being in a doctor's office, she signed the paper after scarcely a glimpse and returned it to Stevens.

I stared at her. She obviously *didn't* understand. Why did Stevens ignore this reality? My mother hadn't heard enough, she was worn out and confused, and s*he didn't understand.* Guilt assailed me. I wanted to take it all back. I was wrong. I suddenly knew it. Rita was wrong. This had to be done. Mother had to get off the road. But it wasn't up to me. It wasn't my responsibility.

I sat in shock, aghast at my mistake, while Stevens questioned Mother for a few minutes about her memory. Almost by rote, I brought up the "person in white" who "got in and moved Mother's checks around on the table."

Stevens asked Mother, "What makes you so sure it wasn't you? How do you know it was someone else?"

Mother said, "The front door was unlocked."

"How do you know you didn't leave it unlocked yourself?"

"Well. I can't know that."

Thus ended Stevens' exploration of the subject and any attempt to help Mother with her dementia. The doctor just trundled on to the next subject. "Someone should live with you. You shouldn't be living alone."

When Mother with her usual obstinacy rejected that notion, insisting no one was needed, I stared at the two of them as if watching an accident. Did Stevens *then* attempt to work with Mother, help her understand her need for live-in help, show Mother some way to face her Alzheimer's symptoms and deal with the turbulent emotions her condition set off? The psychiatrist who specialized in geriatrics treated Mother like a child, then turned to me, the parent. She instructed, "Your mother shouldn't be living alone."

My voice sounded as incredulous and incensed as I felt. "Yes, I know. We've discussed this. She doesn't want anyone there, I don't know where to find such a person, and she doesn't want to pay for something she doesn't want in the first place. Maybe if she didn't have to pay, she'd consider some kind of help." I waited for Stevens to offer the list of services for which I'd been searching. I still expected something!

However, my challenging stare and angry tone brought out her android self once more. Her shoulders again stiffened and she blinked furiously. A moment later, collecting herself, she shrugged offhandedly. "I'm sure the government offers some kind of program that will help you. Or you could call some churches."

Wow. Could you be less specific? Could you be less helpful? The government? Some kind of program? Some churches? Great! "Well, I've called every place I could think of, and I haven't found help yet."

"I'm sure there's something."

It doesn't happen often but even stupid words failed me.

The rest of the visit remains a forgettable miasma of my dumb shock and her clichés and other manifestations of incompetence, inadequacy and insensitivity. It still astonishes me that, regardless of my desperation, I could have possessed one tachyon of belief that she still might help.

Ruthie's Story

A week later I encountered Ruthie again at the market. Her story was heartbreaking. "I called my sister yesterday to see how Mother was and talk to her." Ruthie's sister cared for their mother at the sister's home in Mississippi. "My sister said, 'Ruthie, she won't know you. She doesn't know us anymore.' I just talked to her two weeks ago!" Ruthie had responded. "'She knew me two weeks ago. What happened?'"

"What did happen?" I asked.

"My mother's sister died last month. People with Alzheimer's have to avoid stress. The doctor told us stress was the worst thing for her. She doesn't know us now."

"Oh, Ruthie, I'm so sorry."

***

Stress! How many times had Mother and I discussed it? Even before her dementia began, her frantic searches through the house for mislaid objects was accompanied invariably by the exclamation, "I think I'm going crazy!" (Her dementia never resulted in similar words.) But Mother herself knew stress was unhealthy despite her inability to control it. She was the one who first told me about its effects.

"Stress is just like throwing battery acid on your brain," she quoted the first book she read on brain health. Now I frequently quoted the words back to her. "Stress burns out your short-term memory."

"Is that so?" she responded with interest.

In fact her brain book had inspired her to obtain more than supplements. She purchased several audio relaxation tapes and she taped similar meditations from the radio. But these tapes, we discovered, posed unexpected limitations. One day when she'd been frantically seeking a vanished book, I asked in a mock scolding voice, “And did you play one of your relaxation tapes?”

“Well,” said she. “I stood there for ten minutes looking at them. But I couldn’t decide which one to use. I was making myself so nervous trying to decide that I just gave up.”

“Let me get this straight. You were making yourself anxious trying to decide what relaxation tape to play to reduce your anxiety?”

“Yes.”

We both laughed. The event became a standing joke between us. Eventually, she misplaced the entire set of relaxation tapes.

***

Hoping to help her focus, I made a tape for her myself, a two-minute job based on my own meditation practice. I put in a lot of suggestions for slow, deep, calm breaths. “Imagine you are inhaling all the goodness in the universe. You are bringing the goodness of the universe deeply into your lungs, inhaling it into your every cell, slowly, deeply, a golden light, a golden goodness, and now you are exhaling the old ...Slowly, deeply,” and more in that vein.

“It’s just wonderful,” she told me. She played it while she dusted, washed dishes and sat outside on the deck. Because it was short, she could get the gist with a brief pause to listen. She never had to stop whatever she was doing to lie down and pay full attention, thus losing time, or more time; her time was always vanishing along with everything else. But at least she was listening to a soothing image even if she wasn’t actually practicing it, and whenever she went into flurries of anxiety about mislaying something, I reminded her about my tape, and she played it. Sometimes she actually did stop what she was doing, lie down and listen. Even after she mislaid all her other relaxation tapes, she managed to hang on to this one.

When the "break-ins" occurred, she drank kava tea, went to bed and ran my little meditation tape over and over.

But until Ruthie told me her story about the terrible change her mother had undergone, neither my mother nor I had realized quite how severely stress could accelerate the progression of Alzheimer's. When I repeated Ruthie's story to Mother, I advised, "Play my tape more."

"I will!"

But, obviously, she'd need more help than that.

More Lunacy

Ruthie had given me exactly the kind of information I'd sought from the Alzheimer's Association and Mother's doctors. Now that Mother and I knew the true peril of stress, reducing it in Mother became, as she named it, "imperative." But a professional could do a lot better than me teaching her to relax at stressful moments. I called Mother's HMO psychology department once more.

"My mother," I stated emphatically to the department head, who again answered the phone, "needs some kind of behavior modification techniques. Someone needs to hypnotize her and implant trigger words she can bring up to reduce her frenzy when she misplaces something or there's another 'break-in.'" I also intended to ask whoever taught Mother these techniques for a referral to a biofeedback program. A referral might force Mother's HMO to pay for the treatment. Mother was game for biofeedback. She'd read a great deal about it and was highly impressed, although not yet enough to pay for it herself.

"Someone will call you back," the psychology department woman promised.

Along with the DMV letter, Mother had signed a form saying that her HMO doctors could discuss her case with me. Unfortunately, the person who called me back was Dr. Stevens. My hope deflated, but in my own programmed haze, my own android reality, I just kept going.

***

This was the first time I'd spoken with Stevens since the debacle in her office. I saw no point in bringing up the DMV issue and her disregard for me by betraying my role in it, but now I believe I was wrong. Had I made her accountable, I might have had some emotional leverage. At the least I would have established within myself my own position of power and not fallen into the passive mindlessness that led to my next, crucial mistake. “I want my mother to see a hypnotherapist to help her with her stress. Will you give me a referral to someone in your department?”

“I do hypno-therapy.”

Oh, crap. “I need to talk to someone who practices behavior modification.”

“I do that.”

“Oh” Deep within me I was asking why she hadn’t offered this service when we were in her office. But I gave no voice to my misgivings. Worse, I assumed that since she was Mother’s psychiatrist before, she was the only doctor the HMO would permit my mother to see now. If Mother didn’t see her, she wouldn’t be allowed to see anyone. It never occurred to me to confirm this assumption. Maybe I was just wearing down, however early in the game.

"Let me take you..." or Lunatics and Androids

"What did you have in mind?" Stevens asked.

"I'd like you to try some behavior modification technique with my mother to reduce her anxiety when she misplaces something."

"Your mother would have to be mentally competent to practice the techniques."

"She is. Would you please try?"

"Let me take you in another direction. Your mother needs someone to live with her."

I shook the receiver as if I could get something more intelligent out of it. A bad habit; it never worked. I put the phone back to my ear. "I'm trying to find someone," I said, carefully enunciating each word as if to someone who didn't speak English. or who had dementia. I was equally careful to hide my returning anger at her. "But the government does not offer any services. I still haven't had any luck finding help at churches—" I could feel my careful enunciation disintegrating as my agitation grew. "For that matter," I continued, "I haven't had any luck with my mother. She still won't agree even to a senior companion. So if you could just help her *now*, if you could give her some behavior mod—"

Stevens interrupted in beneficent, patronizing tones. "Let me take you in another direction. Your mother needs someone to live with her or at least visit her every day for several hours."

I took a beat to gather my inner resources then reiterated that I would try again. "In the meantime, her stress is eating her alive. Can you get my mother some biofeedback training and teach her behavior modification techniques?"

"She would have to be mentally competent."

"How do you know she's not? Why don't you try working with her *once?"*

"Let me take you in another direction. Your mother needs someone to stay with her."

"Yes, but meanwhile, isn't it true that stress burns out short-term memory?"

"Let me—"

"That stress is especially bad for people with Alzheimer's?" I recounted Ruthie's story.

She cut in. "That's a different kind of stress. Your mother needs someone to stay with her."

"But hypnosis—"

"She needs to be competent."

I fumed. "How competent does she have to be for hypnosis?" *As competent as you?* I almost said as antagonism began pouring through my skin like my upstairs neighbor's television volume pouring through my ceiling and walls. "Listen, you're underestimating her."

"Let me take you in another direction."

"My mother needs help *in this direction.* You have no idea of her will, her intelligence, her ability—"

I could almost see Stevens stiffening her shoulders and fluttering her eyelids. But then, as before, she rebooted herself. "Let me take you in another direction. Your mother needs someone to live with her."

I thanked her tersely and hung up, failing from start to finish to obtain from Mother's HMO the help she needed. But upon reflection I counted myself lucky that Stevens refused to help Mother personally. Indeed, compelled by my own selfish need, after that conversation I did everything in my power to make sure Mother never went back to Stevens for anything or ever again spoke to her on the phone. For I realized that, being who she was, at some point Stevens undoubtedly would have clarified for Mother my complicity in, my very initiation of, the DMV letter Mother had signed, the letter which would ruin her last days at home, those days I think of now as the end of her fully human life.

Anticipation

Until now, Mother's friends, our relatives and Dr. Burns all exclaimed how wonderful it was that my mother remained independent. "She still drives herself to the store." "She drives herself to the doctor." When I told Elsa, the church social worker, about the notice Stevens sent to the DMV, she was irate. "How dare she interfere in your mother's personal life?"

I immediately regretted telling her. I'd been looking for absolution! Consumed by guilt, not admitting my part in the DMV paper, I told Elsa about the numerous incidents: Mother's "blind spot," her windshield wipers, the brake lights, the car shooting forward in the garage, the white-gowned figure. I said weakly, "Maybe it's for the best."

Only to Dr. Burns did I confess my betrayal of Mother. Burns said, "It had to be done. Do you want me to be the bad guy?"

I thanked her. Why hadn't I thought to ask her first? I was suddenly sick with this unrealized possibility. Mother frequently had appointments with Dr. Burns, and whenever I called her, she called me back and discussed Mother's situation with me without any written authority from Mother. I could have told her what was going on and never risked Mother finding out the truth. "But it's too late."

I hung up accusing myself. I realized I'd assumed (another assumption!) the notice to the DMV had to come from a specialist: a gerontologist, a neurologist, a psychiatrist. Then my mind flipped toward blaming Burns herself. She hadn't come to mind as an option because she'd seen my mother's mental decline herself and hadn't notified the DMV. A thought struck me. *Was it possible none of these doctors knew the law?*

***

Time passed. No notice came from the DMV. I never brought it up. Mother realized a problem lay ahead but, not yet directly faced with it, she rarely spoke of it. But when she did, she attacked me in anger and agony over her visit to Stevens. "Why did you make me see her?"

My remorse genuine and wrenching, I lied repeatedly. "I had no idea she would write to the DMV. I just thought she'd help you with the stress around your forgetting things. That's why I encouraged you to see her."

After several weeks with no notice appearing, I began to hope I'd gotten off the hook. Perhaps Stevens's notification to the DMV had gotten lost in the bureaucracy. I began to breathe.

But what if the bureaucracy did come down on Mother? As Stevens had explained at our visit, the DMV board would interview her. "If she passes the interview, they'll have her complete the written test and then probably make her take a driving test." How could Mother pass an interview and written test under that kind of, well, stress? And if someone with such power watched her every move while she drove, how easily she could make a serious mistake. And what then, when she lost her license?

I asked myself now what she'd asked me before, when she refused to think about giving up her car. What *would* she do? I had to convince her to experiment with one of the two programs I'd exhumed months earlier while investigating driving alternatives. I phrased my suggestion in the following way: "Let's see how this program works, just for those times when maybe you just don't want to drive."

"All right. I'm willing to try," she agreed, willing to prove how reasonable she was. Perhaps, also, she really did admit to herself, if not to me, there just might be a rare instance when she could use the help.

Alternatives

I called the program called Access to make an appointment for my mother and fill myself in on the details so I could relate them to her. The Access woman told me, "If she qualifies, she'll have to make her appointments twenty-four hours in advance."

"What about emergencies?"

"We can't help you with that."

Well, okay. At least they can take her shopping, to the preplanned medical visit and so on.

"Also, your mother has to be ready exactly on time," came the order.

"Or what?" She'll be shot at dawn?

"The van will leave without her." The woman added, "Our vans have to be back at their station by three in the afternoon." This meant that, at best, Access would pick Mother up, drive her downtown, interview her, presumably sign her up and deliver her home by 2:30.

I obtained a few more unpleasant details. As I hung up, the full scale of pandemonium that Mother's first appointment would entail engulfed me, although not to the degree the actual event would do.

***

Mother could no longer get to bed before two or three a.m. (I called her "my senior delinquent"), couldn't manage to organize breakfast or clothing the night before any of her daytime jaunts, and couldn't get up before noon. Once (finally) out of bed, she inched from room to room on her walker. With her old, ever-loosening hip prosthesis, and the fragile hip bone to which it was precariously attached, she had to take great care with each step to minimize pain and avoid falling and breaking her hip again.

Once these painstaking tours of her morning commenced, she invariably became distracted by some book or an article in one of the papers lying about the house, and stopped to read it. Interesting reading matter had snatched her into another dimension.

Lastly, as she went about her slow, laborious endeavor to get ready for an appointment, she would suddenly become hungry ("I was ravenous!") and have to stop and eat. And eat and eat. And read the paper while she ate and delicately sipped her tea.

Thus her time stretched and stretched, while Time, the objective reality, kept its old pace. Mother made all her appointments for late afternoon and gave herself several hours to get up and get there, but she still never had enough time. I'd made Mother's Access appointment for noon, the latest hour for which I could schedule her. Like all appointments with this organization that Mother would make, early doesn't begin to describe it. And she had to be ready. Or she'd be shot at dawn.

First Appointment

Mother set her alarm for 8:00 a.m. I set mine for 10:00. I called her immediately upon waking and continued to call her every ten minutes, keeping her moving along and aware of the passing time, asking what she was doing now and was it necessary, put that book down, go cook those eggs. Each call found her about three inches closer to being ready, and with each of my calls she sounded more frazzled.

At precisely noon she sat at her kitchen table, "famished!" She'd simply been unable to organize herself to cook and eat more than one egg and was now also disgusted, frustrated, angry that I'd talked her into this, more angry that she'd agreed to it and, having slept very little, exhausted; in short, a wreck. But ready.

Access, however, while imposing a pinpoint timetable for its clients, gave its van a twenty-minute window for arrival. "After that—if the van is more than twenty minutes late—call us at this number." I clutched the scrap of paper on which I'd written the number while Mother and I waited for the van. I tasted bile from my own anxiety, thinking about everything that could still go wrong.

For instance, they would call her when they arrived. But what if her phone went out today? Or, as occurred with equal frequency, what if she knocked the phone, which at the moment sat next to her on the kitchen table, off the hook, and didn't notice? What if she'd knocked it off the hook while hanging up from my last call—as so often happened? I couldn't call her and find out without risking her doing it with the new call.

At ten after twelve she called me. "They're not here." Ten minutes later she called again, depression added to her collection of distresses. "They're still not here." Her anger had leapt a few notches higher as well. My own abdominal somersaults were blurred by their increasing speed. I was about to call Access when they called me. "The van is out there, but your mother's line is busy," a woman said.

"She just called me to say you weren't there, what should she do. You must have reached her just as she was dialing me. Let me call and tell her to start out."

"The van is parked on her street. The driver is waiting."

"I'll call her. Just tell the van to wait for her."

Mother's phone rang. Great good fortune! "They're there. *Go.*"

She hung up to gather her purse, coat, walker, keys, at her slow pace, while I called the program back. "She's on her way."

"The van will only wait five minutes." The woman's uninflected tone sent fresh tension crunching the back of my neck. "She can't make it in five minutes."

"Then the van will have to leave."

"But it can't!" My tension grew. "She has to get down a few steps and take a long walk over an uneven, cracked, cement walkway to the street with her walker."

"Then the driver has to see her leaving her house."

"But he can't!"

"We have our rules."

"But her house isn't *on* the street. There's a house in front of hers. It blocks the view." I tried to explain. "You can't see her or her house from the street, and she has to walk very carefully or she'll fall. He has to wait for her." Mother had gone to so much trouble, she was already so depressed and worn out from the ordeal; besides which, she would need this program if the DMV did contact her, test her and pull her license. I simply couldn't let these people leave her behind now. "This is a service for the disabled. *She's disabled.* She can't do it in five minutes!"

"Then the van will leave."

Stupefaction pried my mouth open far enough to let a truck roll through it. Had a plague of androids infiltrated Earth? Or maybe the pod people. She'd never make it. "He has to wait!"

Heart hammering, I called Mother's neighbor at the house in front of hers, and quickly explained. "The van is in front. Can you please run out and tell them she'll be right there? Make them wait!!!" He went out and spoke to the van driver, stalling him until, more than five minutes later, he pointed Mother out as she became visible from the van's point of view, frail, stooped over her walker, snailing along the walkway.

My stomach remained clenched until she was safely aboard the van. Then suddenly someone else was in charge of her. I realized this was the only time in the last few years I was freed from the responsibility and worry of watching out for her. Relief made me feel a hundred pounds lighter. However, the ordeal was not over.

Only now did I let myself consider what the Access woman had further informed me that I hadn't allowed myself to take in. Along with making the pick-up appointment time twenty-four hours in advance, hours too early for Mother, she also had to set the return pick-up time twenty-four hours in advance.

From the standpoint of Access it made sense. How else could they construct a schedule? But how could my mother determine when she'd finish shopping or how long a bank transaction would take, let alone a doctor's visit? I could see her waiting around for the van for twenty minutes or longer, in the winter chill or blazing summer heat, when she was exhausted from whatever chore they were picking her up from. But even this was not the final constraint. I was also warned, "She can only carry two grocery bags."

Two grocery bags? *My mother?* I'd denied the significance of this restriction when I heard it. But while I waited for Mother to let me know she'd signed up and was home, the full impact hit me. I pictured the entire cartful of grocery bags that Mother normally amassed on her shopping journey from store to store. How many days of trips would she now require to bring back all her food and sundries, two bags at a time?

At two she called to tell me she'd qualified for Access and was signed up. "Good," I said, then promised, "I'll find a better program. I'm sure we can work this out."

"Well, I'm glad you're sure," she sneered, said good-bye and went back to bed for the rest of the day.

What Mother Knew and I Didn't

Another round of frantic calls later I discovered that the church where Elsa worked had a van that would take her shopping and a car that would pick Mother up for an appointment, wait with her and then bring her home. This was better! However, the church van also only permitted its riders to bring home two grocery bags and this van too would turn into a pumpkin if it didn't get back to its station by 3:00, which meant they too had to get Mother home by 2:30. Just as with Access, she'd have to start all her church-sponsored trips in the morning. To widen the boundaries of possibility, she could also obtain a few meager taxi coupons every three months.

Tears soaked my face while I scrambled through my mind, trying to work through the limits of each service and put them together—a logistical nightmare. If we timed everything exactly right, the Access van would pick her up and take her to a store. There the church van would get her and deliver her to the next store, where she could fill as many grocery bags as necessary. Then she could call a cab to take her to the final store (waiting on her walker in front of each store for each ride, with her bag-laden shopping cart).

She'd transfer her grocery bags from cart to cab to store shopping cart, into which more bags would accumulate, and call a second cab to take her home. Or else she could just make three or four trips a week. Or something. The fact was, no matter how elaborate the itinerary, mixing and matching services, her entire life would revolve around doing errands.

"If I can't drive, I'd rather be dead," she'd told me, her friends and the whole family. She'd known. Now she repeated it. In fact, she'd probably be dead in the first weeks of a program like that.

And now, a few months before the date set for Mother's finally unavoidable hip surgery, just as her true transportation dilemma became clear to me, the DMV notice arrived. Her interview was scheduled for one week before her surgery. My wildly impulsive feeling in Stevens's office, that I'd made a terrible mistake, became more pronounced. If no doctor took responsibility for her driving, why did I think I was supposed to do it? Having seen the driving alternatives available to my mother, my regret became as hysterical as hers.

A Common Experience

"Why did you do it? This was all I needed!" Sitting at her kitchen table, the DMV notice in one hand, her telephone receiver in the other with me at the other end, Mother burst into tears of hysteria and despair. Every conversation would suddenly veer into her upcoming DMV trip and my role in it, small though she thought that role was. "Why?" she wept and demanded of me. She had all she could do getting from room to room and day to day.

Ashamed and in anguish, I reiterated my lie. "I only thought she would help you with your stress. I never dreamed..."

"Of course not." All at once she was soothing me. "It wasn't your fault. You didn't know what she'd do. How could you?" Then in the next moment, "Why did you make me go see her? Why, why?" She wept and wept.

One evening I sat on my apartment house porch, head in hands. My neighbor Nanette, out walking her little white dog, stopped to ask what was wrong. I told her what had happened, Stevens naming me as the one who'd set it all up, Mother not hearing her but still knowing too much. Nanette, a heavy-set blonde in her mid-fifties, came over with her dog and sat beside me.

"That's exactly what happened to me when I took my husband to a psychiatrist at—" She named a university medical center. "We were sitting there in his office, and the doctor *told Jack* I'd said I didn't think he should be driving. So the doctor said he was going to inform the DMV. They'd probably take away Jack's license. Jack was livid."

I said, "For all the things my mother forgets, she never forgets I'm responsible for this."

"Neither did Jack. He always remembered and blamed me. In court, when we were divorcing, he tried to kill me with his cane. I had to have the police escort me to my car."

My mother continued to alternate between blaming then comforting me, and sinking deeper into misery. "Driving is all I have left. What will I do?"

All she had left? But she was so busy, interested in so much! But the car alone, I realized at last, gave her freedom and independence; and with that, her self-esteem, her very identity. And now the DMV review date approached. The very existence of that appointment, with its racking threat of confiscating her license, was crowned by the horrific journey it demanded. She'd have to drive from Echo Park to the immensely, almost mythically, far-distant city of El Segundo, where the review was scheduled to take place. "Why did you do it?"

What could I tell her? My betrayal had destroyed those remnants of peace she might otherwise have known before her operation and whatever might come after. I prayed Mother would die before she found out the truth. *Please don't ever let her know my role in this,* I begged whatever benevolent divinities might exist in the universe. That prayer became more frequent and fervent as her review date bore down upon her. Then, on another front, her mind began its great leap of improvement. It looked as if she might resume living alone safely, and driving safely, for years.

This is where my thoughts turn again to fate.

Declaration

As far as I knew, no one had ever beaten Alzheimer's. Indeed, unlike with Mother's cancer, nothing seemed to help her despite months of trying this and that. The Aricept the neurologist had prescribed to slow Mother's Alzheimer's produced no side effects. But she'd been on it for two months at the highest permissible dose along with some supplements, and still we saw no evidence of mental improvement.

Yet one night she called me to make her declaration. "I just want you to know. I've decided to lick this." She knew I'd understand "this" meant the Alzheimer's. "I've made up my mind. I'm going to do it. I just wanted you to know." She sounded determined but equally as if she were trying to convince herself.

"Well..." I didn't want to discourage her. I also possessed genuine hope along with the desire to aid and abet. I wanted to be convinced. She did have a history of beating the odds. Coming back from the dead. Mother bore a spirit of impossible resurgences. "If anyone can do it," I replied, "you're that 'anyone.'"

And so she got busy in her old style. She read everything she could find about nutrients that support brain function and brain longevity. She found exciting studies featuring phosphotidylserine and other information on gingko biloba, of which many people were aware. Soon she'd culled together a whole group of supplements, including phosphotidylcholine, Huperzine A, bacopa monniera extract, gotu kola, DHA, DHEA, DMAE, L-glutamine, acetyl-L-carnitine, lethicin—and more.

The next quandary became how to get them all down.

Certain formulas included most of these products in one large pill but in very low doses. Or she could take each of these myriad, diverse supplements separately in high doses. On the one hand, there was a hopeless plethora of pills, a too daunting task. On the other, choosing the one-pill formulas, she literally came within a breath of choking to death a couple of times on some horse-sized tablets which, she decided thereafter, to forego.

In the end she just mixed and matched on a day-to-day basis as an act of faith. Holistic medicine rarely produces immediate results. Her new collection of brain pills still showed no apparent benefits after a month—unless the brainstorm she suddenly had resulted from them: Mother's brainstorm was the qi gong machine. She'd used it in the past and achieved astonishing results for her pain, swollen legs and an enlarged lymph node. Why couldn't it help her brain now?

***

The qi gong machine consists of a black box about a foot long, a foot wide and half-a-foot high. Into this machine you plug a long, black cord that is attached, at the other end, to a "transducer." The transducer looks like a telephone receiver except that one end has a handle. When you turn the machine on, you hold the transducer against the part of your body that you want to help. The transducer produces a gentle pattern of vibration that generates "infratonic" sound, which in turn produces the qi, or energy.

The FDA just approves the machine for reducing pain. But when Mother had slept holding it atop one of her painful groin lymph nodes, she'd wake up in the morning with more than the pain considerably diminished. The swelling in her leg had gone down. Then a couple of years ago she developed a swollen lymph node in her neck. In anyone else the swelling wouldn't have been significant. But with Mother's history of lymphoma, the doctor insisted on removing the node.

Two weeks before her operation was to take place, Mother started sleeping with the transducer resting against the node in her neck. A few days before the operation, she went to see the doctor for a final check-up. The node had shrunk so much the doctor cancelled the operation.

Now, mere weeks before her hip operation, she started placing the transducer against her head as she slept. Pillows kept it in place. After the first week I saw a glimmer of change. She abruptly remembered where she'd misplaced something. Ordinarily, she would have looked frantically until she found it or, more often, didn't. This time the memory simply came back to her out of nowhere. To both of us that memory shone as a small but glorious light that awakened within us a nascent hope.

A week later she did something even more unusual. After finishing writing checks for her bills, she made herself sit at her desk until she'd put everything back where it belonged. "I was afraid if I came back later without having put it all back in order, I'd never be able to find anything." She both recognized and acted on reality.

"Wow, bravo!" I'd begged her over and over to put things away when she finished with them for this very reason. (I was also concerned about more "intruders," although I never said so.) "You actually saw what you needed to do and on top of that, you had the mental discipline to do it. You weren't able to do either one just a few months ago—not for the last few years." I surmised, "It has to be the machine, at least partially, in combination with the supplements."

"It has to be," she, too, believed.

"It was rather brilliant of you to think of it. I guess you still had a few brain cells popping off."

"I probably did." She laughed. Her old sense of irony, always integral to her personality but submerged for a long time by her numerous distresses and symptoms, was returning.

Several days after that, sitting at her kitchen table, Mother announced to me on the phone, "I had no idea what confusion I'd wreaked here! All my files are in total disarray!" She sat there for the next four hours, commencing the prodigious task of reorganizing them.

"This is fantastic!" I said.

"It's like a fog is lifting," she explained. "I must be better."

"You are, you are!"

About this time she had an appointment with Dr. Burns, who also noticed the change. She detailed for me on the phone what happened in her office that day. "This is the first time in quite a while I've felt we were having a conversation. I used to tell her something and she wouldn't respond to it. She didn't take it in. She talked about her concerns but she couldn't hear me. This time she did and she responded to what I said. We talked to each other. It was a two-way street."

Of course, progress did not run in a straight line. A couple of nights after Mother's visit to Dr. Burns, she misplaced something important and reverted to her old ways, frustrating herself in a frenetic and fruitless search. When I called to say goodnight about one a.m., she'd only just given up, exhausted and weak, ravenous and dispirited. Lacking the energy to put any kind of meal together, she had sat down with a plate of raw broccoli over which she poured a bottled salad dressing. When I asked how she was, she admitted her relapse.

"You know what's depressing?" she said.

"What?"

She said, with a heavy sigh, "That I'm better."

We erupted into gales of laughter. We wailed until the tears ran. At incongruous moments throughout the rest of our conversation, we broke into fresh spurts of feverish hilarity.

But she *was* better. Perhaps it was only a brief remission. Or perhaps her symptoms had never come from Alzheimer's. But whatever the source, if she'd been able to continue with her qi gong machine and supplements, if she hadn't needed the hip operation right then, or if the medical system had worked as we had a right to expect, she might have recovered her mind regardless of her trip to the DMV, that hellish journey which, just ahead, one week before her operation, would in a ghastly way add further proof that her mind had improved.

The DMV

The DMV had scheduled Mother's review to take place in the El Segundo office. She'd told me when she received the notice, her tone more resigned than accusatory, "I called them. They won't change the location." I'd dismissed her attempt. I wasn't worried. That couldn't be right. El Segundo posed a staggering drive from her home in Echo Park. If she took the freeway and didn't get lost, she'd make it in an hour. But she only drove the freeways now once a year, on the familiar path to her health conventions. Driving to El Segundo on surface streets at her super careful crawl, watching every sign, making sure she had plenty of space to make any turn, possibly getting lost, would take my mother a lot longer. Moreover, it was June, LA was broiling and her car had no air conditioning.

I would take care of it. She must have talked to the wrong person or people. They simply wouldn't force an eighty-six year old woman facing a major operation a week away to make that kind of drive.

Based on this assumption, I didn't start calling the DMV to change the location until two weeks before her appointment. I phoned her local DMV for two days. When I finally got through the busy signals, I told the man who answered, "I'd like to change my mother's review location to your office."

"I'm afraid we can't change the location of an interview."

"Well, the thing is, my mother never drives that distance anymore. It isn't representative of her driving. She'll arrive a total wreck. The stress will make her sick, and you still won't know how competent a driver she is if they test her after that kind of drive, especially in the heat."

The DMV man explained, in turn, "The competency hearings only occur in seven places in California. El Segundo is the closest to her."

"Seven places in the whole state?"

"Yes."

I wondered silently if they were deliberately making these hearings so difficult to get to because they didn't want someone with a potential liability to pass the tests. "She has a major operation coming up one week after the date of the review. She can't cancel the operation. If she has to drive that far in the June heat, she'll look bad at the review and be sick for the operation."

The DMV guy said, "Try the El Segundo office. Tell them the truth. Maybe someone there will help you."

I called El Segundo. This time the line was busy for four days. By the time I got through and then reached the right person, I was getting anxious. The review date was a week away. Was it really possible they'd give her no reprieve?

Yes.

I pleaded—her age, the operation, how unrepresentative this test would be.

"This is the way we do it. There are no exceptions."

I hung up, appalled and then galvanized. El Segundo! It was out of the question. I called all my friends, her friends and Elsa's church. Someone had to drive her there. It was simply ridiculous to think of her making the drive herself. Surely someone would help her.

But as I made the calls, my desperation grew and my fear for her scaled higher. No one I spoke to could rearrange their schedule to accommodate that long drive, the wait and the return, on such short notice. I'd delayed too long reaching out for help.

A flood of remorse and anguish engulfed me. The only way I could help her now was to call AAA for directions. I requested a route that included street names along the way. "I also need the numbers of the blocks so she can judge if she's missed one of the major streets. Also, I need every turn, all the way from her house to the El Segundo DMV office. Please—no unidentified forks in the road." I typed up this highly detailed strategy, bussed it to her house and tried to convince her not to go. Now it was Mother with whom I pleaded. "You can go after you've recovered from the operation."

"What will happen if I don't go now?"

"They'll take your license. But you can reapply later and show them you can drive. After the operation, while you're recuperating, you'll have time to study for the written exam and make sure you know it. You don't need to go now."

"Yes, I do. I'll pass the test," she asserted with confidence. "I have to keep my license."

"Even if the review board passes you," I pressed, "they'll probably make you come back after you've recovered from the operation and take a driving test."

"How do you know? Maybe they won't."

"But they probably will. That's what the DMV guy told me. They usually do. If there's any question. And the trip to El Segundo is so long, you'll be exhausted. It's so hot. You'll be much more likely not to pass the board in the condition you'll be in." I'd been so afraid that she'd injure or kill someone else, and what if I didn't try to stop it? But now, in the very act of going to the DMV, she could have precisely the accident I'd feared.

Moreover, her potential victim, the victim I'd been so worried about, was only a theoretical person. I massaged my temples, thinking feverishly that if society wants its mentally or physically defective drivers off the streets, maybe society should demand its taxes be used to provide workable, dignified alternatives to such people when they have no family members to drive them around. Otherwise, I thought, if it's Everyone for Himself rather than We're All In It Together, if we're so intent upon a mythology of self-reliance, then let other drivers and pedestrians rely on themselves to get out of my mother's way!

Through this interior emotional outburst, however, I argued, "If you wait until after the operation, I'll have time to find someone to drive you. I'll find a driver. I promise. You won't have to drive yourself there."

"I don't want to go into the operation knowing I've lost my license." She was insistent, unrelentingly stubborn. "No. I have to go. There's no question."

At the last minute, the night before her interview, her adamant position softened. "Do you think I should go?" she queried, childlike. Or perhaps it was a shy, hesitant return of her judgment, further evidence of her improving mental abilities. But I was too demoralized by my guilt to advise her. I'd tried to control the situation before, recruiting Stevens's help, and it nearly destroyed Mother emotionally. Now I just said, "It's up to you. You can still do it after the operation. I'll find a driver for you."

"Well. I don't want to go into the operation worried about this. If I don't go to the review, they'll definitely take my license?"

"Yes. But you can get another review. You can get your license back afterwards."

"Well. I'd better go."

And so the following day, in the blasting June heat, she drove for over three hours to El Segundo. She told me afterwards, "I gripped the steering wheel the whole way."

The Long Journey

Within her house she watches every step. Hanging on to the wall or furniture here and there, she pivots, switching from one walker to another when she passes through the narrow doorways of the old house.

Out on the street, beyond the familiarity of her house, she moves ahead step by even more excruciatingly vigilant step until, finally, the curb. "Oh my god, it's too steep! It's too high! What will I do? How will I get up, get down?"

She parked in the DMV lot and walked all around the building looking for a handicapped entrance. *Creeping along, she scans the ground for ruts over which she might stumble, glancing up and around sharply for danger from cars, casting her eyes to the building and looking for entry.*

"There was no handicapped entrance," she told me afterwards. "There was no one to ask for help." *Stress concentrates in her eyes; her shoulders and hands are tight with tension and fear as she clutches her walker.* "There was nobody at all in the parking lot. Finally, after I-don't-know-how-long, someone came out of the building. They told me I'd parked on the wrong side of the parking lot."

She feels weaker and weaker, from exhaustion, anxiety and the heat waves undulating up from the pavement inferno.

"I got back in my car and drove to the other side of the building. I walked all around the building again, on that side. I couldn't find a god-dammed handicapped entrance on that side, either. I was ready to cry. Then in the far distance of the lot I saw the, you know, the square, the thing. Oh, you know!"

"Kiosk?"

"Yes."

So she ambulated all the way over to the kiosk and asked the woman in it for directions. But she'd been walking around the lot for over an hour. Her appointment was for 4:15. Starting from her house at one o'clock, she had gotten there in time. But the woman in the kiosk said, "It's ten after five. The DMV office is closed."

Mother labored back to her car. The return trip took more than three hours. She got lost, stopped at several gas stations for fresh directions and finally recognized where she was. When she got home, it was after dark. She called me and then, drained, she lay down, too tired even to eat.

Proof

All her life she got lost going everywhere. Now every second on the road to El Segundo she'd been terrified of getting lost again, terrified of being late, terrified of going into the strange building and facing the tribunal, then terrified of not getting into the building, and finally afraid of getting lost and not getting home; all those hours of astronomical stress, in the pounding June furnace, and she drove safely the whole way there and back.

She'd been an excellent driver all her life. It would come back to her. It was coming back already. Maybe there was some luck involved in that this ill-advised expedition ended safely, but maybe it was the final proof. Her health program had put her back on track. *Maybe this is the consummate, the most wrenching irony,* I thought (wrongly). The trip to prove her driving ability proved it, if not to the DMV. The chances of something terrible happening appeared to be no different for her now than for anyone else.

But it didn't matter.

The next day I called the DMV. I told them she'd been there, that the kiosk woman was her witness, but the examiner didn't care. Rules were rules. "She didn't make her appointment."

"Then just do her one favor. *Please.*" I implored the woman I was speaking to not to pull Mother's license until she went for the operation. "Just let her drive one more week." I didn't reveal that Mother intended to do that anyway. I simply didn't want her to get caught at it.

The next day she couldn't get out of bed except to eat a few bites of food. She called the orthopedic surgeon and tried to convince him to postpone the operation. She had no better luck with him than either of us had had getting a closer location for her DMV review. The surgeon informed her, "We have an assistant surgeon flying in from Toronto. He's already on his way. There's no way we can put it off." It seemed the convenience of the doctors was more important than the health of the patient.

Mother was furious at the doctor for insisting on the operation when she knew she wasn't ready. But, she added to me, "I'm just as furious at myself for giving in to him. I didn't have to do this now!"

Normally my mother refused to "give in" to her tiredness. She pushed herself (once out of bed) to do housework, write checks, shop, cook, do sundry errands no matter how exhausted she was, and keep appointments (however tardily). But in the week following her trip to El Segundo, she rose from her bed only once, to go shopping, and then she came home and went right back to bed. She'd driven for over six hours to make that review and roamed by foot all over the parking lot for an additional hour, sweltering the entire time. The night before her operation she was still shaky and sick. How, I thought with fear, would she make it through *this* one?

But that was the wrong question. Just at the very moment of her mental ascendancy, when her Alzheimer's symptoms were dwindling and new years of life lay ahead, she could delay her third and final hip replacement surgery no longer, nor what would follow: I never thought to wonder whether she would survive the *rehabilitation*

The suspension of Mother's license came the day before she left for her operation. At least they gave her that, intentionally or not.

Surgery

The night before her operation she got out of bed for the second time in a week and made up for lost time. She fixed dinner, piddled around and stayed up. She read and ate, ate and read; and sat; resentful, sulking, stubborn and still furious she had to have the operation *right now. S*he stayed up till five a.m., making no effort to get to bed or pack so much as a toothbrush for the hospital recovery room or the skilled nursing care facility to follow.

At seven a.m. her friend and neighbor, Robbie, a wildly red-haired, thirty-something, would-have-been hippie who loved my mother dearly, came to pick her up. Robbie helped her throw a few necessities together.

It was a major operation. The surgeons stitched thirty-six separate pieces of bone together onto the new prosthesis while Mother was still a wreck from her El Segundo ordeal. That morning after the surgery, Dr. Burns called me. "She has blood in her stools. We don't know why. We aren't sure where the blood is coming from; and her abdomen is swollen." Mother's blood pressure had also plummeted. "We have her in Intensive Care."

"Are you saying she might die?"

"Yes, I'm afraid so."

Fighting back tears, I threw on my clothes and raced to the bus stop. After five minutes, frantic with the possibility of still standing there an hour later, I saw a relaxed-looking guy in a blue convertible cruising by. I signaled.

I found Mother in the ICU. She lay dazed by the surgery, the drugs and the complications. I kissed her and sat on her bed. I told her everything Dr. Burns had told me except about the possibility of death. Mother appeared as coherent and intelligent as ever. "Thank you for telling me! No one tells me anything except you." She added, "I used to love this place. They used to take such good care of me. But they're not the same. The nurses are cold. They're rough. They don't care. I'm very disillusioned. I'll be glad to get out of here." She remembered how her mother had chosen nursing as a calling. "No wonder people loved my mother so much. It wasn't just a job for her. Her patients never forgot her." But my mother's mother, *that* nurse, was long dead.

The next day, as soon as I could drag myself up, I bussed to Mother's house, grabbed a nightgown for her, a couple of dresses and books and, most importantly, a portable radio. I threw it all into a suitcase, taxied back to the ICU and discovered I'd been wrong about her mental recovery from the operation.

The Trauma, the Drugs

Mother's brows lifted in pleasure the moment she saw the radio. "Oh, how wonderful!" she effused, reaching for it. "This was so smart of you. What made you think of it?"

I smiled. "Could it be because you have a radio in every room including the bathroom playing classical music?"

She fiddled with the little levers and knobs on the machine with growing frustration. I watched her, dismayed. I told myself, *It's the anesthesia still in her body. It's the post-operative drugs. It's the trauma of the operation.* She could no longer remember how to use a portable radio.

Moreover, despite her glasses, Mother was unable to read the tiny print on the radio which labeled the various little switches and knobs. How was this ever going to work?

Taking the radio from her, I located the classical music station and put the headphones to her ears. She smiled with great joy and relief, took the headphones off and again tried to work the radio herself. I showed her how. By the time I gave her back the radio, she'd already forgotten. I showed her again. And then again. And yet again.

A prickle of fear touched me. I dismissed it. *It's the drugs and the trauma,* I repeated inwardly, my new mantra.

She had one, too. "Just show me one more time."

I did.

But she forgot. "Just one more time."

"I can't. I'm really tired. I only slept a few hours last night."

"Please! Just once more."

I showed her. Then she asked me to show her again.

"I can't! I have to go!" Along with not sleeping, it had taken me all afternoon to get up, dress, go to her house and back to the hospital. I hadn't had time to eat. I didn't want to desert her but my sleepless nights made me weak and hunger left me light-headed. I was sitting, barely able to remain upright.

"Just one more time!" she begged and commanded.

"All right. One more time." I showed her. She tried it. I watched her struggle. I plotted to bring her qi gong machine immediately to wherever she went from the ICU.

"Just once more. I'll remember this time. I promise!"

"You can't promise. It's not you. It's not your fault." But her repeated demand was wiping me out even more. I later learned that repetition of questions is a symptom of Alzheimer's. A pharmacist told me, "Drugs can bring out latent Alzheimer's." Not part of the pre-op information. In addition, only recently have I discovered that anesthesia can cause a stroke. Is that what happened? In any case I did know one thing: "You don't have control over what you can remember. Just let me turn the radio on and you leave it alone. Leave the station where I set it."

"What if I want to listen to something else?"

I answered dryly, "Too bad."

I set the station and gave it back to her, watching her resist the urge to fiddle with it. "Then how will I turn it off?"

She had me there.

"Just one more time. PLEASE!"

I glanced out the window toward the approaching dusk, knowing if I didn't leave at once, I'd have to spend more of my emergency money to cab home. My street was too dangerous to be walking the long dim shrubbery-lined nocturnal block to my apartment from the bus stop.

But she looked so hurt, so betrayed and deserted by my resistance to helping her. She needed the radio so badly! I showed her again. And yet again. And again and again and again. In another minute *I* wouldn't know how to use it. I must have shown her fifty times during that half-hour before I exploded in tears, "I can't! I have to go! I can't do it again! I'll come back!"

"Just one more time!"

"LET ME GO!" I screeched so loudly a nurse poked her head in, then left.

Unimpressed by my outburst, Mother rolled right on. "Just one more time!" She verged on tears of hysteria herself.

"No! I have to go. I'm exhausted. I have to eat. It's dark. I have to go."

"Just one more time!"

"I'm sorry! I love you. But I have to go."

I called a cab and started out of her room. As I reached the door, the nurse stopped me to say, "You should take her possessions with you. We can't be responsible for them in the ICU."

Great.

Well, I'd made arrangements to return in a few hours with Suzann, so I felt I could risk leaving the suitcase; it held nothing of real value and I couldn't face lugging it away after lugging it there. But I went back to get her purse. Mother kept it on her bed next to the giant hardback herb book that she had with her because it was already in the ratty black cloth bag that she carried everywhere, attached to her walker.

After the ICU, both book and purse would follow her from bed to wheelchair to bed. They'd never leave her side on this last journey, upon which she'd unwillingly embarked, until in the last week of her life, when she no longer wanted these earthly parts of herself to hold her here. But now, as I reached for her purse, she cried, "I need my purse! What will I do for money?"

"You don't need any."

"But I might need something else."

"I'll bring it to you as soon as you're someplace where they'll watch it for you."

She regarded me in distress as I gently pried the purse from her fingers and hauled it off, practically falling over. Her purse had to weigh fifteen pounds. What the hell did she have in there? If she could have carried her house, discarding nothing from it, in her purse, she would have done so. And would have insisted on keeping it with her every second.

I left her the radio. It was replaceable if stolen, and she needed the classical music, if she could ever get and keep the station. I set it for her a final time and put the headphones on her ears. She sighed with deep joy; the music fed her soul. When I turned back at the door, she'd taken off the headphones. Again, perplexed and frustrated, she fussed with the switches and knobs.

Exiting the hospital I lifted my face toward the fresh night air. I gulped it down. How clear her mind had been the night we laughed hysterically at the pace of her mental improvement! *You know what's depressing?* she'd said. *That I'm better.*

Even the night before her operation, how lucid she was although still debilitated from the arduous El Segundo fiasco. The street-lit dark surrounding me, Mother's twelve-ton purse at my side, I sat on the stone bench waiting for the taxi, and told myself, *This is just temporary. But the sooner she escapes their clutches and their drugs, gets to the nursing hospital and starts back on her supplements and qi gong machine, the better.*

But when she reached the skilled nursing care hospital and I told Mother I'd bring her machine, she instructed me, "*Absolutely not.* I don't trust them. They'll steal it or break it. It's too expensive. DO NOT BRING THAT MACHINE HERE!" I obeyed her although for a long time I didn't trust her instincts about it.

Her machine would survive.

The Night It Rained

I think of the times my mother might have died and didn't: when she dropped unbatlike from the steel bar across the top of her bedroom door and hit her shoulder; when the neighbor caught her, halting her backward fall toward the cement; when the drive-by shooting missed her; when she escaped the couple who wanted her to get into their truck; when her car broke down, as it seemed to do every other month and always at night, and countless, kind people stopped to help her and make sure she got home safely.

Then there was the night it rained. At a familiar intersection on her way home, Mother made a right turn and the steering wheel stuck. "The wheels only turned right!" she narrated to me on the phone the moment she got home. "The car just went around and around in the middle of the intersection—and the rain was pouring—the night was just black—for almost ten minutes."

"What did you do?" My mouth dry, I pictured the surrealistic scene she described. This was exactly the kind of thing I feared for her.

"I kept my foot very lightly on the accelerator. It was harrowing, utterly harrowing! The car drifted in circles very slowly toward the right. Finally it edged over just far enough for me to park at a curb."

"What about traffic?"

"That was the strangest thing. Not a single car entered the intersection. In fact, there wasn't one car at any of the four streets."

"Then who helped you?"

"I was a couple blocks from a gas station. After I stopped the car, I walked there and called the Auto Club."

A week later, arriving home, Mother called me. "I was at the same intersection tonight. It wasn't raining, but it was jammed with traffic. I've never been at that intersection when every street wasn't backed up with cars."

I envisioned her brown eyes widening with awe, horror and the objective fascination intrinsic to her imagination as she went on, "And here it was just like that again, the heavy traffic. Just a week ago there was no one. If my car had done that any other night—" Dread seeped into her voice. "It was eerie, I can't tell you. I sat there about to make a right turn just like last week. It was like a Twilight Zone."

And the week before played in her mind like a simultaneous reality, the night, the rain, the streetlights and their reflection on the street, the anomalously empty intersection, her car going round and round and round—as her story goes around within me now.

One day when my mother was a young woman of twenty, she developed a soaring, mysterious fever. She left work and, rather than return to her apartment, she dragged herself to her mother's house. When the door opened to her knock, she said, "Mother..." and passed out in the doorway. Her mother, the nurse, took care of her and brought her back from whatever deadly illness had struck.

But when my mother was eighty-six, her own mother had been dead for thirty-five years and her beloved husband for twenty. She went into the hospital for hip surgery and afterwards to a skilled nursing care hospital for recovery, and she had only me to protect her.

But my illnesses, driven by my strange retroviral infection and the loud noise and enmity in my apartment that ignited that infection—those illnesses, which once had sealed our reconciliation, would now make it impossible for me to do for my mother what she needed.

The hospital discharge planner gave me the name of a skilled nursing care hospital that would take me over three hours round trip on the bus. "That will be really hard for me to get to."

She replied, "The next closest skilled care hospital that's contracted with your mother's HMO is in Lancaster."

"Lancaster?" It might as well be El Segundo. Lancaster had to be five hours round trip by bus and a minimum of an hour each way by car, assuming I could find someone to drive me, an effort upon which I could never depend.

No, I had to be able to see Mother. And she had to go to a hospital that was contracted with her HMO or she'd pay out-of-pocket, three to five thousand dollars a month, depending on where she went. So she went to the hospital that the discharge planner advised, the only one contracted with her HMO to which I could get; the one to which, if only once a week, Susie, who is helping me now at Mother's house, ended up driving me.

Mythologist Joseph Campbell says that in fairy and folktales, the dragon, who demands virgin sacrifices and steals gold from the city or village, symbolizes "the system." By which he meant the system of power under which we live.

"You have to be there," friends told me, of Mother's hospital. I didn't believe it.

Mother and I were about to become dragon chow.

***

I tell myself it wasn't my fault! It was the system, and the power of the system, and my ignorance about the system, my naive trust in its professional caretakers despite the fact that one after another proved incompetent or worse. With each fresh incident I thought, *This is an anomaly.* I tell myself that you don't know what you don't know until it devours you. And it did.

In my fatigue it all flowed past me. There was too much I didn't see and when I did see it, when something happened right in front of me, I didn't understand; and even when I understood, or to the degree I understood, I hadn't the strength to fight for my mother as hard as the situation demanded.

I tell myself it was the dragon.

But the moment I turn my mind to the past, jagged fragments of memory come hurtling back at me and frantic wings of blind terror beat adrenalin through my blood. *Wrong! You did it wrong! And where is she now? Gone!*

Staring at the redwood deck of my mother's uninhabited house, I remember our too-few visits and tumble into the bleak void of our loving past and my motherless present.

Where is my mother? What happened?

Ten days after her surgery the doctors still didn't know what caused her internal bleeding. But they threw a couple of drugs at her, and in general she'd recuperated enough from the operation to go to a skilled nursing care hospital.

There was no one now to catch her fall.

Book Five

Thin Veneer

2000 to 2001

Meadows

"I can't reach the water!" "I can't reach my food!" "I'm so constipated it hurts and they won't help me!"

I phone the nurse and repeat Mother's complaints.

"Oh," the nurse says cheerfully, "she made a little poo-poo today."

"'Poo-poo,'" Mother later quotes in disgust. "That's what they always call it here. Very professional. Very medical."

I cannot help a small, rueful smile. This is so my mother. Then I call the nurse back to insist, "My mother needs an enema." But the next day she still can't reach the water, she's had no enema and her poo-poo has not improved.

"It won't come out," Mother says, "or it comes out a little. I can't tell you how it hurts." Beside the expected pain of constipation, the effort to push it out puts pressure on her recovering hip and replaced prosthesis. Days later she gets the enema. That's how it goes here, constipation for days and finally an enema, too little too late.

Months later, when Mother's terrible journey has ended, Camilla will tell me, "One of the first duties of a nurse is to make sure the patient is hydrated and moving their bowels." So I had to force them to give her basic care. When I could.

Then there's the phone. "They moved my phone." "I couldn't reach my phone." "They're always moving my phone." But without the phone she can't talk to me, and I am her lifeline. If she can't tell me what's going on, I can't sit on the nurses to do their job. And she needs to hear my voice, my love. Without the phone, Mother is alone.

And what about a patient's other needs, not only her ties to those she loves but to her personal identity—her own soul? "They never delivered my paper." "My paper's at the foot of my bed. I can't reach my paper." "Someone came in while I was asleep and threw out my paper!" "They only gave me half my paper. Someone else got the other half." "Maybe we should just give up on the paper."

"Absolutely not."

Of course it doesn't end there.

"She was shaking out my covers. She just didn't look. My radio fell and she wouldn't pick it up. I need my little radio! It's the only thing saving my sanity." She means the classical music, which, astoundingly, she manages to get pretty often. "She pretended to look and said it wasn't there. She came back half an hour later and I asked her to look again. She found it."

"I guess it just mysteriously re-materialized."

"I guess so."

The inadequacies rain on—backdrop to Mother's excruciating post-operative pain and, perhaps inevitably, in these circumstances, the abuse.

***

Most skilled nursing facilities assign themselves sundry bucolic, beatific or resort-sounding names. There are Villas, Terraces, Gardens; there are also heavenly attributions, Angels or some such. This place I'll call Meadows. She's come here after the hip operation for skilled nursing care and a specialist in physical therapy. They're supposed to care for her while teaching her to walk again with her new prosthesis. When she no longer needs these specialists, she'll go home. I've asked Isela for help, and she tells me her friend Maria can move into the little bedroom and help Mother for a few more months. Maria will charge three hundred dollars a month and will leave when Mother fully recovers and can again live alone. Toward that end, I fight for Mother from the first day.

But my brain torques, my stomach knots, my heart clenches. As her time at Meadows goes on, my tone with the nurses will become more strident, the fights more furious. A mutual antipathy will evolve between us. For no matter my occasional triumphs over their ineptitude, I keep falling behind the gathering realities, the "anomalies," as I mistakenly and repeatedly regard them. "They never come when I call." "They never tell me what's going on." "They treat me like a sack of potatoes." "I can't reach the—the—button—the thing," the call button for the nurse, for emergencies or when she needs pain medication; the call button, which falls between the mattress and the safety bars or rests above her pillow, out of sight and reach.

She picks up the phone to answer my call and her first words, before "Hello," are, "Oh my god I'm in such terrible pain I don't know what to do." This is one of the two dreadful events that bind and blind me. Caught up in each conflict, I keep missing the big picture and losing the war.

Pain

Whenever Mother calls me or I, her, she's in pain. Her pain ranges from moderate to unbearable. The regular HMO doctor who works there is on vacation. His substitute never calls me back. I think of him as Dr. Kafka, author of existentialist nightmares. Dr. Kafka is the invisible authority and Mother is the heroine. *Why am I being punished? I didn't do anything!* I have to save her. Forget Kafka. I call Erika to discuss Mother's pain.

Erika is the nurse practitioner from Mother's HMO who works at Meadows. She, along with the missing doctor, is another of the alleged advantages for Mother being at a facility that is contracted with her HMO. I call Meadows, reach Station 1, hold, and am transferred to Erika's line, which her voice mail answers. I leave Erika a message but I know I'll have to call back later. She won't call me. Meanwhile, I call the facility again, reach Station 1, hold, am transferred to Station 2, and identify myself. "Can you please find Mother's charge nurse for this shift?" The charge nurse commands the treatment nurse, who in turn administers the medication. When Mother's charge nurse finally picks up the phone, I identify myself again and say, "My mother needs more pain medication." This will be the daily routine and I will do it all day long.

They give Mother her pain pill. It's not strong enough and it's too late. You have to stop pain the instant it starts or the pain cycle will catch hold and hang on, despite medication. But either Mother can't reach the call button to let the nurses know when her pain is starting, or they're too busy to come for ten minutes. Today the pain has already seized her and crushes her in its jaws. This is also the routine. But it doesn't have to be.

Suzann, a nurse practitioner, explains to me about the patient-controlled analgesic, or PCA. "This is an IV drip with morphine. The patient can hit a lever and a bag will release a little morphine. A computer controls the drip so the patient can't overdose, but they can start the morphine the minute pain starts."

When I reach Erika later, I request the PCA.

"Your mother has to be competent to use the PCA," Erika answers with a firm touch of patronization, echoes of Dr. Stevens.

"She knows when she's in pain."

"I don't think the PCA will help. We'll raise the level of Vicodin. That will take care of her pain."

We clash over this day after day, each of us pushing our same arguments, while Erika incrementally raises the dose of Vicodin, switches to morphine, incrementally raises the morphine dose until at last, after Mother has suffered six straight weeks of appalling pain, the morphine dose is correct. But the problem of the nurses arriving too late persists, compounded by another nursing problem, which I discover about a week after Mother's arrival at Meadows.

"How is your pain?" I ask Mother first thing, as usual.

"Pretty bad."

"Have you told anyone?"

"Yes."

"When?"

"...A long time ago."

Ten minutes to get through the telephone routine, then I reach Nancy, the charge nurse. "Please tell the treatment nurse to give my mother her pain medication."

"Your mother's not in pain."

This stops me short. Whatever I expected her to say, this was not it. "Yes, she is."

"No. She isn't in pain."

My bewilderment grows. My anger mounts. "What are you talking about? She's in pain and she says she told you."

Silence.

"Have you spoken with her? Did she tell you? Did you ask her?"

"I don't have to ask her. I can see."

"What are you *talking* about?"

Nancy says, "If someone says, 'I'm in pain,' and they say it like they're asking you, 'Pass the salt—'" she mimics a lackadaisical attitude "—would you believe them?"

"If that person is my mother, yes I would. She doesn't show her pain until she's in agony." I try to tell Nancy about Mother's flat affect. "Her back was broken once and you'd never know it if you were talking to her on the phone. There was no smidgeon of pain in her voice."

But Nancy isn't interested. "I'm here, you're not. I can see what's happening."

I feel a low frenzy start to thrum in my chest. "If she says she's in pain, then she's in pain!" I remind Nancy about the pain cycle. She ignores me. We argue for fifteen minutes. Months later I will learn that my mother's lack of emotional expression when her pain starts, her flat affect, is not even uncommon in hospital patients. A great many of them don't show their emotional reaction to pain until it's so bad that they are writhing and moaning. A friend recently told me about the hospital where her husband's gall bladder was removed. He got a PCA. And the nursing motto is written on a wall plaque: "If the patient says they are in pain, THEY ARE IN PAIN AND GIVE THEM THEIR MEDICATION." But too many nurses have no such instruction and seem unable to sort it out for themselves.

Finally Nancy gives my mother the pill. But only today, only for this bout of pain, and already it's too late. Mother's pain is excruciating for over half an hour before she notices any relief at all. She writhes and moans. The cycle has her.

***

I think: *But this is just Nancy. Once I resolve the problem with Nancy, Mother will be okay.*

But this is the kind of thinking you can't afford because each time something new and horrible happens, it catches you off guard. The problem is never just Nancy or Erika. However inadequately administered, the pain medication has inspired in my mother a touch of Alzheimer's paranoia and the nurses' behavior exacerbates it. Mother, burrowing into her newly inspired paranoia, interprets the nurses' apathy as hostility.

"They all hate me," Mother is saying a few weeks into her stay. She increasingly tells no one but me about her pain. Even when the pain starts to get bad and she recognizes the cycle homing in, she fears asking for help. "I don't want to antagonize them." She is seeing hostility in everyone and fears triggering more of it by asking for pain medication, the bedpan or anything else. "I seem to have inspired their hatred." Sometimes she laughs. "Imagine me, the pussycat, antagonizing anyone."

But still I am naive. There's a hierarchy here but it will take me months to understand it. I only imagine I am climbing higher when I call Jill, the Nurse Supervisor, and describe Mother's physical and emotional condition. "Your nurses have to *ask my mother* if she's in pain because a lot of times now she doesn't trust you enough to tell you until she's in utter agony. And you have to instruct your nurses to believe her. Tell them they have to act on what she says because they don't believe her, and their disbelief makes her even more reluctant to ask for help."

"If you're not happy with the care here," says Jill, the Nurse Supervisor, "you can always take your mother elsewhere."

My heart gives a little jump of fury. I think, not for the last time, *Would that I could.*

Jill reluctantly promises to talk to her nurses. Of course she doesn't. I will argue with every single nurse about Mother's flat affect during her entire stay. And as if Mother's horrific pain and the nurses' reaction to it weren't bad enough, during her first two weeks a CNA (Certified Nurse's Assistant) is abusing her, overtly.

Rory

From three in the afternoon until eleven at night, five days a week, Rory is her CNA. "He glares at me," it begins on her first day. "He glowers." I call Nancy, again Mother's charge nurse, and request she remove Rory from Mother's room.

"I don't have that authority," Nancy replies.

"He glares at her," I report.

"He glares at me, too." Nancy responds without concern, indeed, with something of an attitude. She's already tired of me.

"You're not eighty-six and helpless."

"Call Jill tomorrow." Jill, the Nurse Supervisor.

I call Mother back. "I'm going to call the Nurse Supervisor tomorrow and get Rory out of your room."

"Oh, no!" Her old commanding tone but edged with panic, deteriorating toward tears. "No! Leave it go. I don't know what he'd do!"

I don't tell Mother I've already complained to Nancy. I worry she'll find out anyway, but I needn't be concerned. My protest never goes to Jill. Nancy doesn't bother to pass it on.

After eleven on Mother's fourth night there, she speaks to me very quietly on the phone. "In case something happens to me, I want you to know what's going on here." Rory's gone for the day, but she's still afraid. "I'm afraid he might do something…" Her fear hangs in the air.

My chest tightens. "Do you think he might hurt you?"

"He might…"

"Might what?"

"I don't know."

"Let me complain! We'll get him out of your room."

"No, no! I just want you to know."

But the next day is worse. "I rang and rang and rang. He wouldn't come. He left me lying in my filth for half-an-hour!"

"What?"

"And then when he came—" She weeps, helpless, in despair. "He's so rough when he changes me. It hurts!"

"I have to tell someone!"

"No! Absolutely not!"

But I'm uncertain.

"I needed to go! I couldn't hold it. I wet the bed and now he's going to be angry!" She's been there less than a week and already she sounds like an abused wife who leaves the milk out and gets beaten into a coma for it.

And again the next day, "He left me in my feces for hours!"

"You don't need to go through this."

"I don't care. Don't say anything."

"But—"

"No. Don't complain. *Promise me!"*

While I too anticipate Rory's potential retaliation, I do not share Mother's fear to the same degree. I'm more concerned about what Rory is doing to her spirit and might do to her body in his current behavior. "Okay."

I decide I must at least feel out the possibilities of action. Although I'm anxious at the breach in my promise to my mother, at midnight I call Station 2 and speak cautiously to a different charge nurse than on my last midnight call. "Rory leaves her lying in her feces for extremely long periods." I don't say *hours* because I'm not actually sure how long. I can't believe it's really hours, but I trust Mother's awareness that it is far too long.

"I'll ask him about it." Polite but skeptical.

"He's not going to admit it," I effortlessly guess.

"I still have to ask him."

"And when he denies it? Will you at least remove him from her room?"

"I can't. I don't have the authority. Call Jill tomorrow."

Jill, again. Then I start to wonder. What if Mother's right about Rory? I recall all those TV movies about insane caretakers, serial abusers, hospital murderers. I think about my sadistic psychopathic apartment manager, who still deliberately torments me with noise and anything else he can think of to force me to move and leave him to reign without impediment. Would Rory retaliate and if so, how? What *would* he do? I ask the night charge nurse cautiously, "What if my mother says he did something, and he says he didn't. Who are you going to believe?"

Long silence at the other end of the line.

I tell the charge nurse, "Please don't talk to him about this."

"All right."

But Mother escapes him on the weekend and then he's back. How can she get well?

"I'm supposed to be using the bedpan now! But Rory put me back in diapers." Mother reports his last order: "'You've got diapers,' he snarled. 'USE THEM!' He made me go in them twice." Weeping, she adds with an emerging bitterness, "Then he left me just lying here in my *shit*."

Checking the clock, I see it's eleven-twenty. He left twenty minutes ago. "Have you told the new shift?" I ask gently. We can't count on them to investigate for themselves.

"No. I'll just lie here. I don't want to bother them." Always proud, she now refuses to ask for help and be humiliated again by rejection. But surrender to her powerlessness and filth, even for pride, doesn't improve her morale. "It doesn't matter," she adds dully.

"Yes, it does." Whenever her anger and bitterness abate, despair follows, and soon the archetypal Victim takes over. It infuriates Lucy when she talks to Mother. "I told her not to be such a *mouse*," Lucy tells me in anger and disgust.

Grace, with whom I now speak every night, veers between anger at Mother for being a victim, the facility for making her one, and compassion. "She's helpless there. It's just terrible." But other than emotional support, she cannot help, either. She and Sid live in the desert, too far for their own ill, aging bodies to travel to help mother and me.

"I'm going to tell them about him," I inform Mother. "It can't get any worse."

"Oh, yes, it can!" She perks right up, commanding and imperial. "You promised me you wouldn't say anything. I can live with this. I don't know what he'll do!" She finishes in hysteria.

I grip the phone. "Are you afraid *for your life?"*

A pause. "Yes."

It's finally out. Spoken. Acknowledged. This has been my fear, too. It has seemed too far-fetched—I'm as paranoid as Mother. Is it really possible? Yes. But it *is* far-fetched. But it's been two weeks. If Rory remains her CNA, he'll kill her just from his daily, terror-inducing, humiliating, rough treatment.

Perhaps recklessly, my concern for my mother's intensifying misery finally outranks my own fear of Rory's pathology. He's a bully. Maybe he'll just back off if challenged. Anyway, I don't see a choice. "YOU HAVE TO LET ME COMPLAIN AND GET HIM THE HELL OUT OF YOUR ROOM."

After a moment she relents with a hopeless sigh. "All right." I imagine her lying back in bed in defeat, her head turning away.

It takes three tries because the first two times the nurses don't read Mother's chart and thus don't see the order to get him out of her room.

After Rory

While I'm trying to deal with Rory and take care of Mother's physical agony, I totally miss the next, and decisive, the mortal event. On a day shortly after Rory's supremacy ends, a call comes from Mother's charge nurse of the day. "We just want to let you know that your mother has developed a small bedsore on her back." Her tone indicates nothing serious.

"Oh. Okay. Thanks."

What's that? A bedsore. The nurse doesn't sound worried. I picture a small, uncomfortable, raw sore on her back. Like a bad hangnail.

"My sister died from a bedsore." Suddenly I am sucked back into the present, at my mother's house, where I sit in the yard waiting for Susie. I still speak to my Aunt Grace every night as I did from the time Mother had her operation.

"When you told me she had a bedsore," Grace said last night, "my stomach turned over. It was terrible, just terrible. Didn't I tell you at the time? I thought it was the beginning of the end."

I don't remember her saying that. If she said it, I ignored her and then forgot it. After Rory, and with Mother's endless post-operative pain, "bedsore" never penetrated my mind as a serious problem.

"I told you to make sure they were turning her," Grace says. "From DAY ONE!" As I know now, bedsores develop when a bed-bound or wheelchair-bound patient isn't being turned from side to side every couple of hours at the very least to take pressure off their skin. Their skin should also be examined thoroughly and frequently. A bedsore can also develop from dampness, such as lying too long in a soiled diaper. Did Mother's begin with Rory? "They need to turn her,' I said," my aunt continues. "Did you check? Did you do that?" Did I? "Or did you just ignore me?"

I don't know. I'm drenched in guilt. Grace's memory is better than mine. She said to check and I never checked. I never asked one nurse, "Are you turning my mother?" I assumed the professionals knew what they were doing. The Experts. Why was I such a sucker? I don't trust other "experts." "Trust me," proclaim the experts from the nuclear industry. "We know, you don't, just leave it to us." Don't bother your pretty little head. If I thought about it I'd come up with a whole slew of "experts" I wouldn't trust on a bet. Yet it was Grace I hadn't heard. Her sister had needed an operation to dig the infected tissue out of her pressure sore. Her sister died two weeks after the operation. How often *did* the nurses turn Mother or examine her skin for sores? Could I have saved her if I'd asked? Insisted?

Would they have told me the truth?

But Mother wasn't complaining about her lower back where the bedsore was, I think, as I slip back into the past.

***

"My seat hurts," she begins saying. "I can't get comfortable in the wheelchair. My tailbone hurts."

I ask one of her charge nurses to ask Dr. Kafka to find out why her tailbone hurts. I still haven't spoken to him directly.

"He ordered an X-ray," the nurse informs me the next day. A few days later the nurse says, "Your mother has a little arthritis on the bottom of her tailbone. The bone sticks out and she doesn't have any body fat to cushion her there when she's sitting."

"Can you put some cushions on her wheelchair?" I ask, as if the nurse can't work that out for herself, which, apparently, she can't.

"All right."

Two months after entering Meadows, the notification comes: Miraculously (the notice does not include this judgment), Mother is improving. She will no longer require skilled nursing care or skilled physical therapy, and her coverage therefore is about to be terminated.

Optimism lifts my spirit. *Mother is going where she will be happy and get better. Mother will be going home.* Mother is ecstatic. She's come to hate every second she has to stay at Meadows. "When can I go home?"

Finally I can say, "Now."

Out of Meadows...

But now that it's actually going to happen, Isela's friend, Maria, who was to live in the little bedroom and help Mother complete her recovery, tells Isela, "My husband won't let me stay more than eight hours a day." Isela relates this development.

Boom! Crash! What is Mother supposed to do the rest of the time? Mother has to go home! Frantic mode jacked up again, higher than ever, I call wherever I can think of, to find someone else to help. There are less than two weeks before Mother's coverage ends. I'm on the phone eight hours a day trying to find someone for Mother. Aunt Lucy says, "Why can't you stay with your mother?"

"I'm not strong enough. I'd have be able to catch her if she falls, and she goes to the bathroom all night." I don't go into my whole fatigue thing or my weak back or the bussing/transportation problem in Echo Park.

Sharon suggests Catholic Charities. She'd found a woman there for her mother-in-law. "She was wonderful. She really was like one of the family."

Catholic Charities has one person available. Greta, a German, says she'll go to Meadows on Monday and meet Mother. Then, if she is happy with Mother, Greta and I will meet at the house and I'll show her—the disaster.

How will I ever get that little room cleared out *in days?* Yet if Greta agrees to the arrangement, I'll have to. Isela and I will just have to stash in the tool shed all those one-pound tea bags, boxes of supplements, hundreds of Mother's tapes and who knows what else. No time for discrimination.

But Sunday night Greta calls me. "I took another job today."

The dropping elevator lurch thing happens in my stomach. I suppress the shriek surging up my lungs. I start calling around again, asking neighbors for referrals, looking for someone somewhere to help and totally going crazy until, discussing the crisis with several different people, I realize the whole idea is crazy. The limitations are not just mine. No one person could handle this job. I told Linda, the Meadows social worker, about Isela's friend, Maria, who would stay with Mother until she was completely recovered. Linda did not think Mother would ever recover enough of her mind to live alone, but about Maria she was *pleased.* Why didn't she stop me on the spot? One person cannot do the shopping, cooking and be awake literally day and night to walk Mother between rooms and to the bathroom all night. What were any of us thinking?

Social workers will never prove to be of any help.

I call agencies that provide caretakers in the home on three rotating shifts. At one agency the person who answers the phone sounds as disinterested as a Meadows employee, and the other agencies are exorbitantly expensive. I start looking for some kind of facility. Mother can't go home yet.

I feel terrible for Mother; she is so miserable. But also I feel sorry for me. She is driving me nuts. She breaks into my calls and also rings me between them as I hunt for a place for her. "Get me out of here! I can't stand it. I want to go home."

"You can't. I'm sorry. You need someone to live with you, and I can't find anyone you can afford."

"I don't need anyone to live with me."

"Yes, you do."

"I hate it here! You have to get me out of here!"

"I'm looking for another place for you to continue your recovery."

"Well, if you want a mother, you better find it today. They all glower and glare at me. They don't come when I press the buzzer. I holler and they ignore me. They steal the phone. They won't let me call you. They hate me. I can't stand it anymore!"

I'm as desperate to get Mother out of there as she usually is to go; except every second or third day, when she tells me, "Oh, it's not so bad here. The people are nice."

"Nice? *Nice?* Yesterday, they hated you and you hated them and you couldn't wait to leave!"

"Really? Well, it's okay. They're quite courteous. I'm okay."

An hour later she calls in hysterical tears. "When can I go? You have to get me out of here today—I can't stand another minute!"

I call every place anyone suggests, following a trail of signs, possibilities, referrals and counter-referrals. Finally I find the place I will call Oasis. From the moment I first arrive to inspect it, I'm in raptures.

And Into...

Rose, the administrator, a short, plump, dark-haired Russian who speaks fluent English, trots ahead of me over the clean hardwood floors of the wonderful old Hollywood house that comprises her non-nursing board-and-care facility. With assertive steps and an air of care and efficiency, Rose shows me the huge kitchen fridge from which Mother's fresh meals will come. She promises it will include the huge salads I request and, miracle of miracles, freshly juiced produce. Then she leads me to a homey bedroom at the end of the hallway. Here I find more hardwood flooring, pretty curtains, the profound quiet of an old, well-built house, the kind no longer being constructed. Mother will share the room with only one other woman.

I say, "Can I live here?"

Tony, my new upstairs neighbor, who moved in just before Mother went into Meadows, kept playing his stereo and TV and holding little midnight parties, ignoring my pleas for quiet. Now he punishes me daily for my one inevitable, desperate call to the police: he stamps on my ceiling. He really gets off on it. Rat-tat-tat-tat, he stamps, from flamenco style to machine gun fury, from early morning to late night to the middle of the night, whenever whimsy or his frustrations with his own life seize him.

"He sounds like the people here," Mother said during her first week in Meadows when I told her about him.

"Yeah," I agreed. "He'd fit right in. Rory's clone."

***

Mother will stay at Oasis a couple of months, rebuild her strength and finish relearning how to walk. Rose and her staff will give Mother a sanctuary in which she'll find reprieve from her recent torment and rediscover her joy. Then she can go home. And live alone.

I sign the papers with Rose and call Mother. "I'm getting you out of there tomorrow."

"Tomorrow? Oh, no," very definitive, "I can't go tomorrow."

I'm gasping. "You keep telling me you want to get out of there."

"I didn't mean right away!"

I'm incensed. "You certainly did."

"Well, I'm not ready to go."

I raise my brows. I've become used to her gratitude for all my efforts, her daily repetitions of, "I don't know what I'd do without you!" The balm I've needed to keep me going. Oh, well. "I've set it up. I signed the papers."

Her distress immediately escalates. A tearful panic breaks through. "How can I be ready? What will I pack? I guess I'll have to get up at five and pack."

She's still bed-bound except when someone helps her up and holds her as she uses her walker. It takes me a few minutes to at least partially reassure her that the nurses will pack for her and the Oasis van will come for her (one more boon from Rose's home; none of the other residential facilities have one).

Next time I talk to Mother, she is again ready to leave. NOW.

I reject any notion that the deep quiet of that bedroom in the place I call Oasis, or the thought that I can finally get a little respite from taking care of Mother, influences me unduly.

Trance

Today, sitting in Mother's yard, I am thinking that trauma puts you into a kind of dissociative state, a trance in which you float among the visceral realities that should engage you. But as the trauma deepens, you fall back ever farther from the tangible, visible horrors of it and into your earliest modes of thinking and behaving. *Don't trust yourself,* whispered my old ghosts. *Trust Other People. Trust the experts.* You go into automatic pilot over here so you'll be free to cope with unpredictable twists and agonizing turns of the trauma over there. However incorrect the old program, you let it dominate you so that you don't have to think. *Because you can't think.*

And this is the nature, the unassailable paradox, of trauma. To cope with it effectively, you need to be sufficiently conscious to shift your perception of reality when reality demands it. But that shift of perception is precisely what traumatic trance precludes.

Or perhaps it was only I, after all. I just didn't seem able to motivate my brain cells to take the long synaptic leaps necessary for the clear thought that might have revealed the place toward which we surged, or how to avoid it.

Oasis

The biggest difficulty at Oasis appears, erroneously, to be the language barrier. Rose's three assistants only speak Russian, and Rose herself rarely surfaces at the facility, a fact undisclosed during my initial inspection. But the disappearance of Mother's treasure on her first day calls it to my attention.

Starting in Meadows and now at Oasis, from bed to wheelchair and back, Mother keeps her treasures beside her. The ratty, black cloth bag she'd always attached to her walker holds the countless toothbrushes I've brought her, other odds and ends, and her huge, hardback herb book. Next to this bag, her radio and giant purse make quite a crowd on her bed. "You don't have room for the phonc on your bed with all this," I often kidded her at Meadows. "Maybe that's why you keep knocking it off the hook. Can't I please just put something in the closet?"

"No! I have to be able to reach everything," she insisted, her old adamancy incontestable. Over the next months her command would become more plaintive until, finally, she would say of these objects, "This is all I have in the world." But now, on her first day at Oasis, Mother's Russian caretakers move her ratty black bag. Mother is hysterical. "They took it off my bed and they won't give it back! I don't know where it is! I can't make Lyla understand me!"

Rose answers my page that night. "Lyla put your mother's bag in the closet." In the morning Lyla gives it back to her.

A wall TV runs day and night on the living room wall. "If I have to watch television, at least I want to watch channel 28 [the local PBS station]. I can't make them understand!" Rose responds a couple of days later to my message on her page. "There's no way to turn the channels."

"I can't see to read." Something is happening to Mother's eyes. Have her cataracts become worse? "They make me go to bed at eight and the light is so weak. I can't make Lyla understand! I need more light! And Rose is never here."

When finally I reach Rose, she promises to get Mother a lamp. Later in the week, I ask Mother, "Did they bring you a lamp?"

"Yes." She sounds disgusted. I don't ask. But on my next visit I see the lamp. It sits on the mantle on the other side of the room across from Mother's bed where, especially with its low wattage, it's useless to her. I think, Can't *anyone* do *anything* for my mother without detailed instruction? Do I have to do *everything?* But they don't and I can't and Mother's anxiety is mounting.

"They leave me outside on the patio and never check on me!" At Meadows the nurses had left her on the patio until the sun burned her face; she'd begged the nurse who appeared in a doorway to take her back in. "But she just closed the door and left me there." I told them to stop taking her out. But I'm sure the Oasis people wouldn't do that.

"They don't check on me at night. I'm in that room at the end of that long hall. I feel so alone. What if something happens? I'm frightened all the time."

But I think this time she's wrong. I think, *That paranoia again.* Of course they check. This is where she's getting *better.* I plan to bring Mother her qi gong machine as soon as I can get back to her house to pick it up. That will make all the difference.

Then Mother calls me in pain. Rose, who is there for a change, won't give her the medication. Rose has given her a glass of water instead. "Sometimes old people are confused. They ask for pain pills when what they want is water."

"My mother knows who she is, who everyone else is, where she is, and *she knows when she is in pain."*

"I have to see for myself."

"Well, give her the pills and see that way." Rose's lack of perception unnerves me. Have I misperceived *her?* Is my mother just another interchangeable old woman to her, too?

When further language misunderstandings occur, I start thinking something critical could happen that would demand Mother's caretakers speak English. I call the organization that referred me to Rose. The woman there asks, "Do you want to complain? No one ever complained about Rose before."

"No one?" Maybe I'm wrong. Maybe there's no problem. Maybe after Meadows, I'm just oversensitive. Mother's eating well. She's gaining a little weight. She looks less skeletal. She's not getting the promised giant salads but she's getting salads, she's even getting fresh juice once a day. I've seen it there at her meal when I arrive at dinner or lunch; I go a few times a week for about half-an-hour. I can reach Oasis with one bus; it's only half-an-hour from me.

They also give Mother a daily shower. Grace tells me, "None of the other homes offer that." And Rose or one of her assistants walks Mother up and down the driveway forty minutes a day—thirty-five minutes more walking than she got at Meadows.

"This is what I need!" my mother tells me. She might be bitter or angry about Rose one minute, but in the next she's telling her, "I love you! You're wonderful. Thank you so much!" I share Mother's ambivalence about Rose but trust wins out. Most impressive, I have observed that pink flushes Mother's cheeks. "You've got color on your face."

"Oh?"

I think, *She's already better here.* I decide not to complain about Rose.

Then the new thing. "I think I have to go back to the hospital."

But I don't believe her.

She repeats this as endlessly as she's begun repeating everything, part of the Alzheimer's. I, as endlessly, reiterate, "The doctor at Meadows"—Dr. Kafka, but I don't insert this—"released you. He doesn't think you need skilled care. And an HMO nurse sees you here every two or three days. Plus, you're seeing Dr. Burns next Monday. I know the language barrier here is a bear, no pun intended."

She doesn't laugh. She doesn't even get it.

"But soon you'll be able to go home." I am determined that soon she'll reclaim her mind and enjoy puns again. Rose gives her the supplements I've brought over, but I have yet to get to Mother's house to pick up the qi gong machine. But when I do, she *will* be okay.

The next event seems to validate my optimism about Oasis. I discover that when Dr. Kafka, the Meadows/HMO doctor, determined Mother no longer required skilled care (and thereby caused her coverage to be terminated), she still had the bedsore on her lower back, the one that the Meadows nurse had called me about several weeks earlier. Now Rose tells me that it periodically opens up. "The nurse showed me how to clean and bandage it. I showed my assistants."

"Oh, good," I say, a blithering idiot, knowing nothing, questioning nothing, thinking, *Rose is really on top of things. She's learning what to do from the nurse, and she is conscientiously making certain Lyla and the other caretakers know how to do it when she's not there. Mother really is in a good place. I can let go of the reins a little and trust someone else to take care of her.* You get a positive belief, a hope, an ideal of something or someone, and without sufficient evidence or clarity you continue to act as if it were real.

But of course that's not the whole thing.

I conclude Rose cares after all. I really believe it. But also I have to believe it. So that I can take care of my own needs.

The Wheelchair

My immune system has crashed for the third time. It wasn't coming back to normal, but I've located a doctor at Cedars who gives me magnesium and Vitamin B shots; and I have to find another apartment. The quest has again become urgent. Along with the threat from my plummeting blood counts, one of my fellow tenants has become very scary.

A month ago Ron moved in upstairs and one unit over from Tony, he with the machine gun feet still banging on my ceiling. Ron's stereo bass *whomps* into my bathroom and culinary cubbyhole, both places in which I spend time. Ron's rage toward me since I finally had to call the police about his noise has driven me back to the great apartment hunt. "Drop dead," says Ron whenever he sees me. Or, "I wish you'd drop dead." Or, "If you died, I'd feel—let me think—GLEE." He glowers into my street-facing bay window when he passes it and, if he's outside and sees me exit the apartment house, he pauses to glare balefully at me. Another Rory clone. Like Mother before me, I am now afraid for my life.

But the drugs, pain and stress have taken their toll on my mother. She demands and implores me to come see her more often. She doesn't understand that I sometimes have to balance, or choose, between our needs, or that I cannot make the right choice. There is no right choice.

"You only have one mother," one friend says.

My Cedars doctor says, "You have to take care of yourself. If something happens to you, who will take care of *you?"*

Or of her? I think.

Or is that just my excuse?

I explain to Mother I'm afraid of Ron and of my crashing immune system. I have to go to Cedars. I have to find another apartment. I have to get out of bed, although I can barely move. But she does not hear this. Today my mother knows only how lonely she is, how helpless. She no longer understands anything except her own misery, including this: "I'm in pain." I lose track of how often she tells me. It isn't every phone call or even every day. Or is it? "I hurt."

Yet it seems not to be as bad as in Meadows. She never moans and writhes when I speak with her on the phone or visit. It never occurs to me that she might undergo excruciating pain at other times and forget or not bother to tell me. But I call Burns, who prescribes a higher dose of morphine.

Mother's pain is in her hip or back, she's not sure which, only that it's getting worse. Despite more morphine, days later Mother reports something else. "I have a pain in my asshole." Deliberately vulgar because she's so angry. She hates her helplessness, her continuous pain, the way everyone treats her because she's old and because her once-resolved memory problems have transmogrified. Now she needs people to keep repeating everything and she can't retain any of it. "Tell me again why I can't go home." And she's angry because I'm not there and not getting it. She is in pain. I'm not hearing her. She says she's in pain and even I am not there for her.

Because this time I think she must be wrong. The pain can't be that bad. It can't still be going on. We finished with all that. It was finally under control when she left Meadows and now she's in good hands. Finally. If something were really wrong they'd tell me, Rose, Dr. Burns, the nurses, someone. The home health care nurses check on Mother at Oasis every two or three days.

True, I can't get the nurses to call me and report on Mother's condition after a visit. I leave messages for them at Oasis. Lyla, at least, understands that much English. I leave another message at their central office. PLEASE CALL ME! Naturally, they don't. But nurses see her often and although each time it's a different nurse, which triggers my doubt, I think, *They keep records. They can keep track of any changes through her records.* I think, *And Mother's pain can't be very bad or she would be screaming.* But the truth is, I can't bear to hear about it anymore. So I don't. She's falling apart, but I can't see it.

***

"I think I have to go back to the hospital."

The first time I visit her at Oasis she has a bandage on her upper arm just as she did at Meadows, for the same reason. Her skin is so fragile it breaks and bleeds when they help her out of the wheelchair onto the walker. On my visit a week later, a second bandage has appeared, this one on one of her swollen legs.

Since the return of her cancer twenty years ago resulted in the swelling of her lower legs, the lymphedema, she's had to keep her legs raised whenever she sits. This minimizes the swelling and prevents blood from accumulating in her lower legs. She always has to be careful. Any tiny break in the skin of her lower legs can lead to infection. At home all her chairs are piled with fifty pillows to make herself comfortable as her legs rest on the chair seat opposite.

Mother's first nurse at Oasis arrived while Mother and I were on the phone. The nurse came on and told me she was ordering a semi-reclining wheelchair for Mother. A couple of days after that, Mother and I were on the phone when she suddenly exclaimed, "Oh, the guy with my wheelchair is here!" and hung up. But now as we visit in the patio a few days after that, I watch her shift around in severe discomfort. Lyla places pillows at her feet and tries to raise her legs onto them but Mother gasps in pain as the movement stresses her hip. "No! No!" Suddenly it hits me. Mother's in a wheelchair from eight in the morning until eight at night. What happened to the semi-reclining one, the one she needs to lift her swollen legs?

I call Burns, who orders another semi-reclining wheelchair, which doesn't arrive. Burns tries again. While

Mother waits, pain increases in her hip/back despite the larger morphine dose, and "the pain in my asshole is terrible!"

Life always brings back your particular difficulties in a new way. As Rita would say later, "Sometimes it doesn't look like a snake. This time it looks different. But it's still the same snake." I don't think Oasis is the same snake, although Mother attempts to tell me. "I think I need to go back to the hospital." But I don't hear her. It's the same snake. But I am still in a trance.

The ER

These people at Oasis care about her. I'm certain of this on my next visit. Mother sits at the table eating her dinner. They give her what she needs! I tell Mother, "I have to go."

"Oh, no. Can't you stay longer?"

"I have to find another apartment. I have an appointment to look at one." As Mother sits at her dinner table, I explain again about Ron. "I'm sorry. I'm really afraid of him. He's always telling me to drop dead. I have to keep that appointment."

"Oh." Her expression closes up into loneliness. She withdraws into the abandonment that has become her life.

And the shameful truth is that I do have time to stay another ten minutes. But I'm falling over from fatigue, I'm seconds from audibly voicing the scream of madness clawing constantly at my throat, I feel battered and beaten up in every cell from the noise and antagonism in my apartment building; and the dining room television here, attached to the wall above the dining table where Mother sits, roars above us like an angry god, reverberating agonizingly in my head and through my every shredded nerve. Everywhere I go loud televisions pursue me, clinic waiting rooms, the post office; and loud bass seems to thunder from every car on the street.

"I'm sorry," I plead. But it's not as if I'm leaving her in Meadows! And as soon as I find myself a new home base, I can expend all my energy on my mother. But I have to use my little last scrap of strength to find that place. If I leave now, I can walk slowly to the bus stop breathing the air in the quiet street outside. I can gaze glassy-eyed at the large, graceful trees and unique, old, attractive apartments and houses. I can pull myself together; whereas if I stay here one more minute, I'll just fall apart. "The guy is crazy."

"I think I have to go back to the hospital."

Or am I being selfish and a fraud?

I kiss her good-bye. As I head for the door, I feel her watching me go. I feel her eyes on my back. I can't stand it. I'm nearly out the door when, compelled, I glance back at her.

She has pushed herself away from the table. But she's not looking at me after all, or anymore. She's given up on my staying. She's let me go, forgotten about me. She's never said anything to me about her own exhaustion, she's never said she needs to lie down, and it has never occurred to me. Quite the opposite. *Wow!* I keep thinking. *She's up all day. This must mean she's recovering really fast. She needs to get up. They told me so at Meadows. And here she is, up.*

But now she sits in her wheelchair, her head back with nothing to rest it against. Her eyes closed, her face is slack and drawn in an agony of suffering and what, in retrospect, I will recognize as an unbearable weariness of body and soul. She's still in the regular wheelchair, the reclining wheelchair has yet to arrive, and her legs are down twelve hours a day. She can't get comfortable, she can't rest, and the pain in her hip/back/rectum is unrelieved. No one will save her, love her. She can't stand it. *I want to die,* her body screams, her slack silent face begs. *Please just let me die.*

But Rose has said nothing about Mother not doing well, and wouldn't she know? Isn't she here all the time? Or at least some of the time? Rose knows about old people in Mother's situation; and *Rose is here right now and thinks everything is fine so it must be.*

I leave, but I will never forget how Mother looks.

The following Monday Rose takes her to see Dr. Burns, who also does not call to tell me anything is wrong. But three nights later, at ten, my phone rings. "Her other leg opened up," Rose reports. "It was bleeding a lot. I called the paramedics. They bandaged her leg."

At Mother's HMO the next morning, where Rose has taken her in the van whose existence had once impressed me, the Emergency Room doctor discovers Mother has an impacted bowel. This is “the pain in my asshole.” “She’s also dehydrated,” the doctor informs me on the phone.

Then the calls start. The ER doctors and nurses call me incessantly, demanding I remove Mother. They’ve cleaned out her bowel and need the bed.

“I’m looking for a place for her,” I retort. I’ve lain in my own bed with the phone book, calling all day. But all the nursing care hospitals are full.

I finally find one with a free bed for Mother. I’ll call it Orchards. It’s a temporary stop until Meadows has a bed for her. For I’m still operating on the advice of the discharge planner at the hospital where Mother had her operation: Unless Mother pays $3,500 or more a month out-of-pocket, she’ll either have to return to Meadows or go to Lancaster, the two closest hospitals that are contracted with her HMO. Meadows is still preferable to sending her to Lancaster.

If I’d understood as much about Meadows as my mother did, I’d have made sure she went elsewhere, close enough for me to visit. She’d just have to pay the money. She would have been glad to do that. But I didn’t trust her judgment, and I was trying to save her money for when she went home.

In Greek myth Prometheus is the God of Foresight. But it is his brother, Epimetheus, God of Hindsight, who will rule here, along with the God of Pain. And of Death.

The Mystery

At Orchards the nurses push Mother in a wheelchair to their phone at the nurses' station. (It takes four or five days to get a private phone installed. She won't be there long enough to start the process.) She tells me, "I screamed all night for pain medication. I'm going out of my mind from the pain."

My stomach starts churning. What's going on? When did her pain get like *that?* When we hang up, I call back the nurses' station, asking for her charge nurse. "Why didn't my mother get pain medication last night?"

"We needed a prescription from the doctor. There was no doctor here last night."

"Why didn't you call him?!"

"We don't do that unless it's an emergency."

Stunned, I tell the charge nurse to call the doctor immediately and get him to order the medication. The next day I receive a call from Dr. Ryan. It turns out he's the doctor who was on vacation, and whom Kafka replaced, when Mother was in Meadows. Ryan covers both Orchards and Meadows. As I absorb this, fresh shock strikes. "The nurses told me that when your mother arrived," says Ryan, "she had a bandage on her lower back. When they took it off, they found a Stage IV Pressure Sore. Do you know what that is?"

"No."

"It's a kind of ulcer. A wound. A Stage IV Pressure Sore is a serious wound."

"She said she was screaming from the pain."

"Yes, it's very painful. I'm ordering that she be bed-bound. If she sits, she'll disturb it and prolong the healing process."

"How long do you think that will be?" I ask.

"Three to four weeks. She'll be better off at Meadows. It's contracted at her HMO. Orchards only HMO-approved; I or another doctor can only see her once every month or two there. At Meadows a doctor will see her three or four times a week." Because Meadows is "contracted."

"Meadows says they'll have a bed within a week," I say, trying to take in this appalling distinction.

"Good."

The next day I hop on a bus. I haven't spoken with my mother since the doctor ordered her bed bound because she can no longer get to the facility phone and they can't bring one into her room. I've barely begun to comprehend the seriousness of her wound. But as I enter her room, she looks shrunken, and the first words out of her mouth are, "Thank god you're here! I'm literally going out of my mind from the pain."

I can't believe it. I race into the hall for a nurse. Is there no end to what my mother must go through? I do not yet realize the full, dreadful nature of Mother's pressure sore. But I see the shift that has occurred from "I hurt" and "pain" to ghastly pain, mind-destroying pain; and I feel, along with a rush of suppressed tears, a rage toward the ER. Where else could it have happened?

Yesterday I told Rose what Ryan said about Mother's pressure sore. Rose exclaimed, "We gave her a shower that morning. There was nothing on her back. Nothing!" Yet when Mother arrived at Orchards a day-and-a-half after entering the HMO Emergency Room, she had a bandage on her back and this horrendous pain. Between Oasis and Orchards, that is, in the ER, she had to have gotten the pressure sore.

For months, as I discover the nature of a pressure sore and watch Mother descend into stupefying agony, I will believe the ER was responsible.

Hitchcock and the Rose Revelations

When I get home from Orchards I again call Rose, who cares so much, and describe what I've seen. Rose tells me, "You know we can't take her back the way she is. You just touch her, her skin breaks. She's falling apart. And it's 'Pain! Pain! Pain! Pain! Pain!'"

I pause. This statement jars me. It doesn't surprise me exactly, yet something in me staggers. Each time I think about these words over the next months they will jar me more deeply, a little quake getting bigger and more violent with each jolt until finally my thoughts come to the epicenter.

The entire time Mother was at Oasis and she complained about pain, I told myself, *If she has anything seriously wrong, the nurses would tell me. Dr. Kafka would not have dismissed her from Meadows in the first place. Dr. Burns would have said or done something. And Rose, who sees my mother every day and whose profession is caring for elderly women, would have noticed and told me.*

I'd trusted Rose above all. I was responsible. But she was there. I did hear Mother tell me she had pain. But she told me with her flat affect. I didn't recognize the signs. Now it turns out that Rose heard "pain, pain, pain, pain, pain" *all day long.* And she said nothing to me.

Rose now adds, "She needs round-the-clock care."

"I know." As I say it, another thought surfaces. My mind starts reeling forward and backward about the semi-reclining wheelchair.

Mother wouldn't have gotten this agonizing wound in her back if she hadn't gone to the ER, but she wouldn't have gone to the ER if her legs hadn't opened up and bled; that is, if she'd gotten the semi-reclining wheelchair. I ask Rose, "Do you know what happened to the wheelchair Mother was supposed to get? It arrived and then it wasn't there."

"Wheelchair?" she says. "What wheelchair?"

"The semi-reclining wheelchair the first nurse ordered."

I can sense Rose shrug at the other end of the line. "I don't know anything about a wheelchair."

"The first nurse ordered it."

"I don't listen to the nurses. They all say different things. I just listen to the doctors."

"Oh," I say, as if reality were not commencing to suspend itself, time winding down to a point of infinity. I realize what must have happened. The wheelchair guy told Mother she couldn't get the new wheelchair unless she returned the one she was using. She got confused, disappointed, sent back the new one and kept the wrong one. Lyla had no idea what was going on.

And Rose?

I'm too stunned to conceive the question that Camilla will ask me in our long conversation months later about the whole string of events, in the conversation that will send me whirling back in time, into this period, and plunge me full force into the lowest depths of my grief. Camilla will say, "Did Rose call the doctor to find out what she had to say about conflicting nursing instructions?"

My voice will be dull as I reply, "Rose never mentioned asking any doctor anything."

***

Until my conversation with Camilla, I will, like Mother, believe in Rose's warmth, and continue to love her for it. But Camilla will disillusion me. "You can't get a Stage IV Pressure Sore in two days. Hortense couldn't have gotten it at the ER."

"I love you," my mother told Rose, when she wasn't angry, anxious or cynical about her Russian caretaker. "Thank you so much!"

Between bouts of my own cynicism, I thought, *She's giving Mother what she needs. My mother is getting better!*

Relieved and with incipient elation, I'd observed Mother's pink cheeks as she ate dinner that night. But eventually the truth will dawn on me. Rose and her staff walked my mother up and down the driveway forty-five minutes a day. The pink in my mother's cheeks was *sunburn.* And despite her sometime love for Rose, Mother also sensed the truth. *They don't watch me... I think I have to go back to the hospital...*

Decades ago, in a Hitchcock story Mother and I watched on television and discussed afterwards, a man lies on a slab in the mortuary. Everyone thinks he's dead. But in fact he's alive and conscious. He can't speak because he has some medical condition that prevents him from being able to move a muscle. But in voiceover you hear his thoughts, his desperation, his terror and horror as he listens to the morticians discuss the autopsy the coroner is about to perform on him. He's frantic. But his case is hopeless. The story ends as a tear leaks from one of his eyes and they realize he is alive.

"Can you imagine anything more horrifying?" Mother had exclaimed. "To know you're going to be tortured because they think you're dead and you have no way to tell them you're not? I can't imagine anything more terrible!"

She told me what was going on. But she couldn't make me hear her.

A bed becomes free at Meadows and back she goes.

It can't, I think, get worse. Or much worse. But I do not yet have the faintest clue about pressure sores, or Meadows. Or the edge of the cliff at which we've nearly arrived.

Return to Meadows

"I need you here!" she cries out with my every call as soon as I get the phone installed. "When are you coming? You don't know what's going on here. They torture me!" But, like the first time she was at Meadows, I can only see her when Susie drives me over. She's been there a week before I get my first opportunity to visit.

As I enter her room, which she shares with two other elderly women, I pause in the doorway, staring at her. Mother lies on her back, eyes closed. The color is gone from her face, which is again skeletal. Her hair looks whiter and thinner; her skull shows through. She didn't used to look eighty-six. Now she looks older.

Dr. Ryan has called to tell me, "Her pressure sore is infected. I've ordered a low-pressure airflow mattress overlay. It'll help alleviate her pain and allow the wound to heal." I see at the foot of her bed a spaceship console-like contraption with winking lights. To what other world is it taking her?

I think her eyes are closed but as I approach closer, they open and focus on me. She must have glimpsed or sensed movement through half-closed lids. The instant she recognizes me, her older face becomes animated: it twists, breaking into a thousand wrinkles of hysteria and agony. "Where were you? I needed you! I needed you!" Tears rush down her face along all the old and new wrinkles.

I recoil with guilt. I've called the facility every day. "How is she?"

"She's doing fine," her nurses say.

Now I lean over and kiss her. I take her hand, which is icy. I massage it, and smile, and try to explain that I just couldn't get here sooner. But all my mother understands is that she needed me and I wasn't with her.

Looking for a chair, I realize that a trash can stands next to her bed. It holds her discarded bandages. "This is what they think of me." Her negligible gesture at the trash can is dismissive. "This is what I am to them. Trash."

I explain the can needs to be there to hold the hazardous wastes her infection generates. She doesn't care. This is what they think of her.

I've never seen her like this. I talk and talk, trying to engage her, to make her feel better, to make me feel better, but nothing touches her bitterness or depression. When Susie comes to pick me up after an hour, I walk out to the hot parking lot to meet her. It's a hundred muggy degrees, late summer in LA. I tell her I'm going to stay longer. I'll use some emergency food money for a cab home. I can do this if it's not too often. I watch Susie's little red car drive off.

When I get back, lunch is being served. Mother perks up a little. "The food here isn't very healthy but at least it's tasty." While she eats, we talk, and I sort her mail. Just as during her first stay at Meadows, Robbie, her red-haired friend and neighbor from Echo Park who drove her to her surgery, brings her mail here, the halfway point between us. I go through it, setting aside all the health come-ons and other junk mail to toss out. When I come across Mother's absentee presidential ballot, I just assume she won't vote. She isn't up to it mentally or physically. I say nothing, dropping the ballot into the junk pile.

The phone rings. It's Lucy. "Alexa is here," Mother brags, sitting up a little more, showing some spirit. "I'm starting to feel like a human being for the first time."

As always, Lucy hates the phone; their conversation is brief.

I tell Mother my latest lousy-apartment news. She's interested again. I explain my decision to vote Green in the upcoming election. I give her my reasons. She listens to my criticisms of the Democrats. "I'll have to think about that," she says; weirdly, I do not discern the dichotomy between my dismissal of her ballot and her intention to vote. Who's losing her mind here?

Then the meal is over and she lies down again. The weariness comes back over her face. “When can I go home? It’s like a prison here.” Then she adds, as she’s done on the phone, “They torture me!” And just at this moment, the treatment nurse comes in with two women CNAs. Mother mutters that the prison guards and torturers have arrived. I move my chair to let them through.

Killer Wound

Mother speaks metaphorically. I am about to learn the metaphor is apt. The CNAs walk to one side of her bed, the nurse to the other. I watch the nurse cut strips of tape and attach the tops of them to the edge of Mother's bed. Then she asks the two CNAs to turn my mother onto her side so Mother's back faces her. **"AHHHH!"** Mother screams the minute they touch her.

I freeze in horror. The CNAs move Mother onto her side and hold her there. "**AHHHHHHHHHH!"** Screaming in agony, she grips the bed bars while the treatment nurse gently strips off the old bandage from the wound on her lower back. Tears flood down Mother's cheeks. **"NO! NO!"** she begs. But the nurse peels off the old bandages while Mother, with her icy hands, clutches the bars of her bed, sobbing and screaming.

My mouth falling open, I watch the outer bandages come away. They expose a burn-like redness across most of Mother's lower back. My breath turns so shallow that I might have stopped breathing.

"**AHHHHHHH!"** Her tears stream, torrential. "**NO! *STOP—"*** She continues to cry out, her agony intolerable. ***"NO--!"*** The nurse removes the bandages from the wound itself and I can't move. I stare as the last bandage comes off, revealing to me the wound itself, and I see for the first time what has happened to my mother.

I am looking at a hole in her back the size of a child's fist. The red meat of her flesh forms the circular wall of the hole. Her red flesh looks like the raw meat in a supermarket, in cellophane-covered packages, except for the putrid yellowish pus-like infection that rims the surface of the hole. The hole goes clear to her spine. As the treatment nurse gently cleans the wound, Mother clings to the bars of her bed, screaming, ***"NO, I CAN'T STAND IT! I CAN'T STAND IT!"***

Suddenly I'm released from my shock. I jump up and run over to the side of the bed. One of the CNAs moves aside for me. I hold Mother, I grip her to me and kiss her head, her soft white hair, as she clings to the rails of the bed and her screams of agony dissolve into small, hopeless whimpers of unbearable despair.

She has to go through this twice a day.

When it's finally over and the nurse and CNAs have gone, Mother says, "I'm glad you saw that." She's recovered better than me. I still can't breathe. She told me she had to go back to the hospital. Once here, she told me she needed me. Once more I haven't heard. She told me they torture her. They torture her.

Dr. Ryan has said it will take her wound a few weeks to heal. Is he crazy? This will take months. I think, Will she have months, if she is *here?*

Downhill

The moment I get home, I call Dr. Ryan about Mother's horrifying pain. He sounds shocked, as if (though he won't admit it) the nurses have told him nothing about it. "I'll raise her morphine for when they change the bandage." But I have to call him almost daily. It's not just the bandage-changing. "Oh—oh—oh—" Mother convulses in agony as I listen helplessly on the phone. "It just comes in such terrible waves—ohhhh!" Compassionate, Ryan keeps ordering higher doses of morphine for the day plus an extra dose for bandage-changing and her physical therapy, which is equally excruciating. She only manages to stand for minutes. Ryan also writes on her chart that the nurses must check her every hour to see if she needs a pill for her "breakthrough pain."

Mother also undergoes unnecessary suffering because some nurses don't have bandages prepared for the wound-cleansing. I watch one of the CNAs turn Mother onto her side and hold her there. Then the nurse removes the old bandages. And only then, while Mother waits, panting between screams of agony, clutching the bars of the bed, does the nurse cut new bandage strips.

"Why aren't you ready?" I demand. Every second Mother has to hold that position means horrible suffering.

Matter-of-factly the nurse returns, "I didn't know what I'd find. I don't have time to read everyone's chart first."

"Well, read my mother's!" But she won't and I can't make her.

However, I do manage to cut off another abusive CNA at the pass. On one visit I see Georgia (I note her name tag) go behind the curtain separating Mother from the woman next to her. Behind the curtain the woman patient screams. I hear no soothing words from Georgia. I report this incident to Jill, the Nurse Supervisor, who responds in distaste, "Oh, I know that patient. She always screams. Just worry about your mother."

I think, *Mother could have ended up like that without me.* I think, *That patient has no one to fight for her.* I think, as I have begun to do lately, *That could be my own future.* But I have to try to waylay further enmity between Us and Them for Mother's sake. I back off.

But two nights later around eight, while Mother and I are talking on the phone, I hear a woman, whom I shortly ascertain from the charge nurse is Georgia, order Mother, "Shut the hell up and go to sleep." I report this the next day to Jill who, annoyed and a bit angry, says, "You'll have to talk to my boss." She transfers me to Nina, the Director of Nursing, the next rung up the hierarchy. Nina, however, refuses to believe me. "I'll have to investigate," says Nina. "But this kind of thing doesn't happen here."

"I heard it."

"You weren't here," she reminds me.

"Neither were you," I retort. Nina had gone home at five, three hours before the incident occurred. I ask her to please remove Georgia from Mother's room during her investigation. She refuses to make that commitment. We argue for fifteen minutes. What's *wrong* here? Despite my best intentions to keep my cool, my rage escalates. She keeps repeating, "I have to investigate." She simply will not commit to getting Georgia away from my mother.

I call back ten days later to learn the results of Nina's "investigation."

"Georgia?" Nina is puzzled. "Investigation? What are you talking about? Why are you so rude when we're doing everything we can for your mother?"

I throw a fit, bursting into tears. "I trusted you! I trusted you!" At the back of my scrambled mind, I think that my anger hasn't provoked any human behavior. Maybe my hysterical grief will cause some guilt. Guilt is good. And it works on her. Grudgingly, Nina checks. Georgia is no longer in Mother's room.

But Mother continues to deteriorate, her Alzheimer's intensifying. The harder I struggle to pull us out of the pit, the deeper into it we sink. One morning I wake up to three messages on my phone, all left between four and five in the morning. "Call me, I have to know you're okay." "Call me! I'm worried about you!" "Call me! I'm getting frantic!"

When I return her calls at noon, the hour at which I begin to function, I speak gently, firmly and wearily. "You know," I say, "I can't call you back at four in the morning."

"Of course not," she agrees, rational to the core.

But another script goes on and on until I'm ripping out my hair. Every time my phone rings I sink into my deepest depression yet.

"Call me," Mother says. "I need to know you can reach me." I call. "Now I'll call you. I need to know I can reach you." She does; she can. But her fear and need are insatiable. "Now you call me." "Now I'll call you. Wait! I havc to write down your number in case I forget it. Wait while I put it in my herb book. Wait! I've dropped my pen! Wait, wait!" Ten minutes while she looks. "What's your number? Wait—I've lost my page! Okay, what's your number? Wait—my pen fell—" "Now I'll call you." "Now you call me."

"I can't call you back one more time!"

She breaks into tears. "All right, do what you want."

I break into tears. "All right. One more time."

We replay that scene until, bringing meager relief, our conversation reverts to a different rerun. "When are you going to get me out of here? When can I go home?"

I beg Ryan for help. He gives her a new sedative. Before her operation she'd taken only thyroid pills. Now she is on sedatives, sleeping pills, antibiotics and anti-depressants.

The new drug is a disaster. "I don't know how to get home! I'm here in Mexico and no one will help me."

"You'll be all right," I assure her, frightened, from my apartment. "I'll help you."

"How will you help me? I'm in a phone booth in Mexico but I don't know where."

"I'll find you."

"How will you find me? I don't know where I am."

"I'll go to the ambassador," I improvise.

"How will he know how to find me?" she cross-examines with her old attorney style, sharp as ever, in her delusion.

"He has contacts," I struggle to keep up with her impeccable logic.

A pause. A new turn. "How can I trust you? How do I know you'll help me?"

"I'm your daughter." I'm in tears. "I'll always help you."

"You're my daughter?" She sounds uncertain.

My tears scald. "Don't you recognize my voice?"

"Well." She reasons it out. "I'm not sure."

"I'm your daughter! I'm Alexa! Don't you believe me?"

More logic, carefully phrased. "You could just be saying you're Alexa."

I call Ryan. *"Change her drug!"*

The next day she knows me again. I tell her what happened. She doesn't remember. "It must have been terrible for you," she exclaims. After that drug, although it is supposed to completely leave her system, hallucinations continue to loop in and out of her days.

Then for about two seconds help seems to arrive. *Deus ex machina.* "The glorious messenger riding comes," sings a character in a play by Bertolt Brecht, who also wrote, elsewhere, "He who laughs has not been told the terrible news."

Ombudsman

The newest social worker, who's demonstrated no competency or initiative to date, has called a meeting with the ombudsman, Emily, a stout woman with short, coarse, gray hair. We meet with the hospital administrator, Wendy, to whom I give a polite nod. An ombudsman! I've never even thought of this. But I recall vaguely from somewhere that an ombudsman is supposed to fight for the patient. Something like that. And so, turning to Emily, I begin to enumerate my problems with Meadows.

But Emily interrupts me, her attitude disengaged. "Have you discussed any of this with the Director of Nursing?"

"The Director of Nursing is one of my problems," I snap, and start to describe my experience with Nina, Georgia, the "investigation."

But Emily peremptorily motions toward Wendy, sitting behind her desk. "Have you spoken with the administrator?"

I turn to look more closely at Wendy, whom I'm meeting for the first time. She is slim, trim and attractive, well-dressed in a neat suit. She spends a lot of time putting herself together and making it look simple and effortless. I'm wearing jeans and a loose top. My hair, a mass of split ends, has not been cut in years.

Wendy does not leap forward to proclaim her shock at the complaints I've managed to get out; nor do I see any compassion for my mother's suffering or interest in exploring our problems. Instead, she sits with her slim, manicured hands clasped on the desk before her, listening politely with an intelligent, business-like expression.

I turn back to Emily, confused. My thoughts run so fast they jam at my throat. *I called the social worker, the nursing supervisor, the Director of Nursing, and the doctor.*

"Why would I go to the administrator?" But even as I speak, clarity begins to stream into in my mind, hosing away the cobwebs and revealing the outdated concepts. It has never dawned on me that I should deal with this hospital as a political institution, not a medical one.

But Emily continues brusquely over my silent monologue, striking up more shock like fire from flint. "I'm just here to make sure you know that your mother's hundred days of skilled care coverage runs out in a month. You need to decide if you want her to stay here or find another place." I stare at her as she hands me a booklet listing skilled care facilities in Los Angeles. "You should start looking now." The social worker nods in agreement, with an intelligent expression of her own.

So much for fighting for the patient.

When I get home I start calling the facilities closest to me. I lie in my bed, the phone on my pillow, as I swelter and melt in the late September heat. It's still over a hundred degrees. Even the television blasting through the ceiling and walls sounds drenched in sweat. An hour into my latest project a particular hospital intake worker tells me, "We can't hold a bed more than five days. I'd be surprised if other hospitals do." My next calls confirm she is right.

Then why did Emily and the social worker tell me I should start looking *now?* Mother won't be leaving Meadows till November. a month away.

A few days later, acting on Emily's accusation of my ineptitude, I call Wendy, the well-appointed administrator, to try to forestall further problems at Meadows while Mother remains there.

My mother had loved the Tarzan books, which she too had read voraciously at one time in her life. From them she often quoted her favorite recurring line, giving a dramatic flourish for coda, "'And the thin veneer of civilization fell from him *like a cloak!*'" Mother's recitation comes back to me when, talking to Wendy, I see at last what lies beneath the very thin veneer at Meadows, thin and more ratty than Mother's cloth bag.

The Dragon

Laying out Mother's problems for Wendy, I begin with her excruciating pain. "I don't think the nurses reported it to the doctor. He was always surprised when I told him how much pain she was in. I think there's a problem with the system—"

Wendy interrupts, "Does your mother still have pain?"

"Not right now, but if the system is broken—"

"Don't worry about the system. Let's just take this on a case by case basis."

Case by case. I take a breath. "All right." I bring up Georgia. "Why couldn't Nina just promise to pull Georgia from my mother's room while she investigated?"

"Georgia? Who's Georgia?"

Startled, I relate the Georgia story, what I heard her say to Mother and then deny.

"I don't know anything about that. I'll have to investigate." No, she isn't speaking with irony. Her tone also makes clear that I'm a real pain in the ass.

Still attempting to deflect a build-up of mutual bellicosity, I install a tone of courtesy into my words. "I thought it was your policy to take a nurse or CNA out of a patient's room if there was some kind of conflict with the patient. When my mother was there the first time and I complained about Rory, he was taken out of my mother's room."

"Rory?" She sounds puzzled.

I'm incredulous. Can she not know about *Rory*?

"Who's Rory?"

She *doesn't* know about Rory!

I start to tell her, but she's on a roll. She pounces. "So you complained about someone else! If you complain about everyone, there won't be anyone left to take care of your mother."

I've been sitting up straight to maintain alertness. This posture suddenly becomes impossible. My body sags with shock. But of course what she says makes perfect sense. Wendy represents the origin and the endgame in one. The disregard Mother endures at the lower end of this political hierarchy mirrors precisely the apathy against which I bang my head at the top.

Phone receiver in hand, I remember my favorite line from satirist Mort Sahl. "You know how you're always appalled but you're never surprised?"

"Is there anything else?" Wendy asks.

"No." I hang up and lie down for the rest of the day.

Yet only later will I truly comprehend the magnitude of what Mother and I face. The people who own Meadows also own about thirty other such hospitals. Other, larger corporations own twice that number and some probably own more. Thousands and tens and hundreds of thousands of people pass through them. Millions. The parents of seventy million Baby Boomers, and the Boomers are the next wave, right behind their parents, all paying collectively hundreds of millions, possibly billions, of dollars. That is the real system. The system of power under which we live. The system of medicine for profit. That is the dragon that devours the innocent and steals the gold of the populace.

***

Within the week Mother's phone loses its dial tone. Like those disabled phones at her house, this one is always having problems. The volume control stops controlling the volume, the long-distance operator doesn't come on so Mother can't call Sid, Grace or Lucy; or there's heavy static.

"How's my mother?" I ask the nurses each day, waiting for the phone people to fix the phone.

"She's fine."

Dr. Ryan has ordered the nurses to check her every single hour for pain. He's written it in Mother's chart to make certain they do it, so they must know how she is. But when after four days her phone works again, Mother has her old, deep, wracking, Atlantis-heaving cough. I call Ryan. He orders X-rays. It's pneumonia. Either the nurses didn't check Mother for pain or they just ignored her cough. *That* cough. Wendy's "next case." I don't bother calling her.

It can't get worse.

Who says?

A new deadline abruptly appears like a rooftop sniper.

Rehabilitation

Orthopedic surgeons don't tell you what can happen when they perform a hip replacement surgery on an older person with an overt or underlying dementia: the anesthesia and pain drugs can cause confusion, dementia and a memory loss that makes recovery impossible.

During Mother's first stay at Meadows, George, the physical therapist, told me, "I tell her to get up by leaning forward and bending her knees, and she leans back and straightens her legs." She could have reinjured her hip, making it necessary to repeat the operation. As it was, she lost her HMO/Medicare coverage twice.

In order to maintain your coverage, you have to need skilled nursing care, which she did. You also have to be able to follow instructions from the specially licensed physical therapist. She couldn't. I wrote the HMO and spoke to people in her HMO membership office, insisting that Mother's inabilities were due to having been abused by the CNA. The HMO restored her coverage.

Now at Meadows again, pain medications control her pain most of the time and damage her mind all the time; and her physical therapy remains agonizing.

"I told her she needs to walk." George, still the skilled physical therapist at Meadows, regards me, his eyes large behind thick coke-bottle glasses. He sits at the nurses' station writing a report. I like him. He is direct and honest.

"But she's in so much pain."

"She still needs the therapy. She needs to walk. She just stands a couple of minutes and quits."

With a sudden flutter of fear, I realize how much time has passed since Mother's pressure sore broke out. George is the one to whom I must address the fresh fear growing inside me. I stand watching him writing something up. I stall. But have to ask what I so don't want to know. "How long until she loses the ability to ever walk again?"

"Two or three weeks."

I inhale sharply. "That soon?" I don't know what to do.

He adds, "She needs to move in bed. Do bed exercises. 'Move or die.' That's what I told her. I had a long talk with her today. But she doesn't want to hear it."

"Someone has to go in there and work with her because she won't remember bed exercises on her own."

"Oh, people help her," he assures me, looking down at his chart.

I stare at him. I talk with Mother day and night. She hangs up to eat, take a pill or when someone has time to help her to the bathroom. But she's never once had to hang up because someone came in to remind her, let alone work with her, on bed exercises.

I don't challenge him. This is my old, strange passivity, the sense of reality floating past. I leave him; I leave my trust and respect behind as well. I go to Mother's room. "You need to do bed exercises."

"Oh, you're right!" she says, and in her old proactive style, she immediately begins to throw herself from side to side on her bed with her upper body. I smile; a small hope suddenly burns.

Since that terrible sedative she has never quite returned from the deeper seas of hallucination. Beyond her panicky anxiety, paranoia, sleep disorder, depression, increasing memory loss and the shrinking margins of mental clarity, dementia has become a permanent factor. If she goes home, maybe the familiar surroundings, healthy food, supplements and the qi gong machine will provide a slim chance for her mental recovery. But she'll need to walk or she'll end up back here or someplace like this.

But by the same token, walking won't save her from such places if she has no mind; and the longer she stays here, the more permanent her mental damage becomes.

But she won't go home. What am I thinking? *Move or die.* I love her but I know that despite my love, I won't be able to call her every hour and remind her to do the exercises. And George was lying. No one here will help her.

She too knows. She tries to shout above the reality, a drowning woman.

"Help me!"

"Help! Help!" she starts yelling, forgetting she holds the call button in her hand on those occasions when it hasn't slipped into the crack between her mattress and bed bars. Most nurses ignore her. A few conscientious ones rush in but she's already forgotten why she called them. "I'm sorry, dear," she apologizes, her fear evaporated at the sight of help. They begin to ignore her, too, and her anxiety escalates. She shouts again.

Dr. Ryan claims the only solution to her anxiety is more drugs. But the drugs seem to make her sleep more; and, when she's awake, she seems more anxious than ever, crying out for help more frequently. The doctor doesn't tell me about the "rebound" effect. At this time I have no idea that eventually many drugs produce the very symptoms they're meant to cure, or mask, e.g., drugs to control anxiety make you more anxious.

I ask Ryan, "Isn't anybody there trained to deal with Alzheimer's patients or old people who feel abandoned and frightened?" Susie has told me that an elderly friend of hers also started shouting for help once he entered the hospital.

Ryan avoids answering. I say okay to a new drug but then I call Nina, the Director of Nursing. "If you do something to ease my mother's anxiety before she yells for help, won't it help your nurses, too?"

"We're doing our best. Why are you accusing us?"

Jeez, lady. Take one of your own pills.

I even call Wendy. Dementia is contagious. I tried a while ago to get the administrator's permission to bring Mother a lamp. Mother's eyes are worse, the fluorescent bed lamp is behind her and when a nurse raises her bed—when she actually gets such help—bringing her to a sitting position to read, she casts a shadow over her book or newspaper. "If they don't kill me first, I'll die of boredom."

Wendy referred me to the maintenance man who expostulated, "The fire marshal! The fire marshal!" I called the fire marshal, we made arrangements and then I called the maintenance man again, explaining the type of lamp that was permissible. "The fire marshal! The fire marshal!" He volleyed me back to Wendy and she, to him. Back and forth I went, trying to explain I'd cleared everything with the fire marshal, but Wendy refused to have anything to do with it and I could not get my message through to the maintenance man, who spoke little English.

I finally gave up, instead bringing Mother a clip-on flashlight for her newspaper and herb book. But she can never remember how to use this flashlight though it's simpler than a portable radio. Now on the phone I say to Wendy, "My mother can't be the only Alzheimer's patient or older person with some kind of dementia in your hospital. Somebody must have come up with a better way to handle them than just ignoring or drugging them."

"We're doing our best."

Then, as my mother would have said, *you'll just have to do better.* I don't say that. Obviously.

When I'm with Mother I hold her hand and gently massage it. This calms her. My friend Barbara tells me that she does the same for her neighbor, who has Alzheimer's. "I stay with him and rub his hand for half an hour. It seems to calm him down for the rest of the day." But I'm only with my mother once a week.

I call the Alzheimer's Association and explain Mother's situation. "Do you have any low cost or volunteer services, someone to visit Alzheimer patients in the hospital and literally just hold their hand?"

"No."

"But that might save her. She just needs to feel someone is there for her—and make sure she gets basic care."

They're sorry. They can't help.

Back on the old telephonic tour I call churches, temples, government agencies, charities. But my strength to is limited; the time to pursue this objective was *before* the operation. With my scant energy and time, I find no place that offers handholding, nurse-monitoring services, which Mother needs with desperate and increasing urgency.

When nurses or CNAs do perform their nursing duties on Mother, they discuss her over her head. "What are you saying?" she asks, demands, pleads. They keep talking. She cries out in tears, "I can't hear you. What are you saying?" The more they ignore her, the more abandoned and frightened she becomes, and the more she screams. "Help me! Help me! Help me!"

My mother has sunk even lower on their food chain. She's gone from being an interchangeable old woman to just another "patient who screams."

"You have to kill me," she tells me. "You have to help me die!"

Innocent

"I want to go home!" the new conversation begins.

"Not yet." I speak gently, from beneath the dark fathoms of a truth I refuse to accept.

"I'm going to jump out the window!" she threatens with determination, on the verge of hysterical tears.

"You're on the first floor." I smile. I try to cajole a smile from her in return. I can't think ahead. I won't. Instead, I try to bring back her spirit, to save her. But for what? She's passed the point of no return. She cannot even remember that she'll never walk again. She'll never be able to live alone and she'll never go home. Then for what kind of life am I trying to help her smile, am I trying to save her?

It doesn't matter. She doesn't smile. She is frantic. "I can't go on like this. You have to help me die!"

***

The trash can still resides beside her bed. Her wound is still infected and so is her urethra from the catheter they've inserted to keep the wound on her back dry. "She pulled out her catheter this morning," says the nurse when I arrive.

"I hurt," Mother tells me in a childlike voice, pointing, "down there."

"You pulled out your catheter this morning."

"I did?"

She keeps losing weight, if that's possible. Her hair, that still had brown in it before her operation, has turned pure white in these hospital months, and her face has a pallor to match. I remember how her skin used to glow, made luminous by all that juicing; and how, after the cancer had been gone for several years and she got lazy about juicing, still all the raw vegetables with which she began each meal including breakfast gave her flesh a subtle radiance. Now her skin just lies across her face, lifeless.

Lucy finally got to see her. It took her over three months. Lucy is eighty-three and in bad health herself. She entered Mother's room, saw my mother and stormed back out to the nurses' station. "My sister's not in that room!" Mother is so deteriorated Lucy didn't recognize her own sister. Which is one of the ironies. Everyone in our family has been concerned that Mother might not recognize *Lucy.* "Do you know who I am?" Lucy asked her. "Of course," Mother said with the new childlike demeanor she has acquired from the drugs and physical and emotional trauma. "You're Lucy. You're my sister."

Now I sit on her bed and massage her cold hands. Her eyes remain half-closed. The door behind me stands open to the busy hallway. The closed curtain on the other side of Mother's bed separates us from the other two patients. Mother and I are alone here, alone in the universe, suspended together in shock, surrounded by its buzzing silence. How did this happen? She defeated cancer—and how close she came to triumphing over the madness and degeneration of Alzheimer's. Indeed, she managed so many dramatic, narrow escapes. How has she ended up like this after all?

And what can she or I do to restore the life she had before this place, a life she might have continued to have, had she not needed the hip operation, or if her "rehabilitation" had not destroyed her? She asks only this one last thing of me. "You have to kill me."

"I can't. I'll go to prison."

True, but not the whole truth. I've concocted a manner by which she might achieve the death she craves, a method by which she might escape. But my throat closes over what she aches to hear, the words that might divulge the action that is, above all actions, irrevocable. I've been thinking about it for weeks, since she first started saying she wanted to die.

I picture myself leaning over to whisper in her ear, "If you really want to die, keep asking for morphine even when you don't need it. Tell them you have pain even when you don't. The morphine might kill you." But I never lean over like that. I'll never get the words out.

But on my next visit, I wonder if I'm a coward.

As I approach her bed she entreats my compassion and faith in her. "They're going to execute me." Worry and fear mark her face, from which her beautiful Hepburn-like features have been wiped away forever. "They say I killed my husband. I didn't! I'm innocent! Do you believe me?"

I tumble once more into shock, a bottomless pit with only brief pauses from one drop to the next.

I recall how, when Mother first came back to Meadows, she called it her prison. She referred to the nurses and CNAs as her "prison guards" and "torturers." But she was speaking metaphorically. Today I affirm quietly, "Yes. I believe you. I know you're innocent." She's gone from seeing Meadows as a metaphorical prison to hallucinating that it is a real one. "I'll get you out of here."

Her hundred days of skilled nursing care ends in one week. But even if it didn't I would get her out of Meadows, whatever the cost. Someone has told me that if her money is put into a special trust, she will be poor enough to qualify for Medi-Cal. They will pay for her hospitalization and then her money, such as it is, can be used by a trustee to make her more comfortable. If the trust thing is incorrect, her money won't last long at the rates hospitals charge and she'll soon be poor enough to qualify for Medi-Cal anyway.

In either case my only concern now is finding a hospital that will take good care of her, one that is at least HMO-approved. At an HMO-*covered* facility, my mother would pay but a doctor would see her three or four times a week. However, I'm still not willing to send her to Lancaster. I still believe the evil fairy tale that Lancaster is the next closest HMO-covered hospital. But maybe I can find an *approved* facility; then at least a doctor will see her once every month, or two. I also want her someplace I can get to more often—without needing anyone to drive me.

***

Once home, I retrieve the pamphlet that the social worker and ombudsman gave me. I go down the list of skilled care hospitals it contains. At each one that I call, I name Mother's HMO and ask, "Are you approved by them?" One receptionist replies to my question, "We're contracted by that HMO."

"What?"

I must have misheard her. She must be wrong. "You mean you're HMO-approved*?"*

"No, we're covered."

I try to process this. She *must* be wrong. This place is closer to me than Lancaster. It's closer than *Meadows.* She tells me again. I didn't hear wrong and, questioning her further, I determine that she is not wrong. My heart thumps like the ceiling stereo. This is a place I can get to on my own. Mother could have gone there instead of Meadows. She could have been there all this time. I could have visited her two or three times a week. They might have helped her keep walking. Their caretakers might have actually *cared* for her. *She might still have a life.* I can't take it in.

But now my mother will need a bed that can become a Medi-Cal bed when the time comes and today they have no such bed free. They won't have one until someone dies.

This is what I find repeatedly in my calls—and learn as well that more of these facilities are HMO-contracted. Mother could have gone to any of these places, rather than Meadows.

But how do I find the best one for her now? At each hospital I ask to speak to the Director of Nursing (DON). I describe what happened to my mother at Meadows and listen to their response. I use these descriptions of Mother's treatment as a kind of testing board. One DON becomes irate on Mother's behalf. I burst into tears at her compassion. A

DON at a different facility says, "It might take us a few days to locate a problem with abuse, but we would." Which at least sounds honest and caring. These two are the best I find. But neither has a bed free for a Medi-Cal patient.

Ultimately, I locate an HMO-approved skilled care hospital about an hour from my apartment. Maybe the place I will call "Haven" will work out. Tony, the administrator, informs me that the nurses specialize in caring for pressure sores. "Doctors who have patients here are surprised at how fast people with your mother's kind of wound heal." They heal, he says, in several months.

"As opposed to?"

"Not at all."

And Mother will see a doctor from her HMO once every month or two.

Even after everything I've seen, it never occurs to me to doubt Tony's promise of good care, to imagine that the horrors can continue to mount.

Even after Mother's death, when I think it is all finally over, I will find myself wrong then, too.

I sign the papers to transfer Mother to Haven. Then I do what I've been itching to do for months but didn't for fear Mother would suffer retaliation. I call the Department of Health Services (DHS) and complain about almost everyone.

Haven

Only in the future will I talk with several people and put together how to find a good nursing hospital: go to each one, check for cleanliness, and ask the patients and their visitors how satisfied they are with the care. If possible, bring a nurse you trust to check out the medical situation. Of course this may not be possible and of course, for various reasons associated with the system, it may not help. But in any case I do not know any of this now. I transfer Mother out of Meadows and into Haven.

For a while I tread my old trail, trusting doctors, nurses, authorities, professionals. They know, I don't, blah, blah, blah. If something's wrong, it's an anomaly. It's the Anomaly Syndrome. The Bad Apples Syndrome. Ignoring my instinct that the whole system is rotten and I cannot trust anyone including myself.

Trauma. Trance. Shock. Exhaustion. My guard is down. My ego boundaries are permeable. My defense mechanisms barely flicker. And so all those strangers and murderers still in my unconscious, all those Other People figures who personify attitudes and opinions that are not mine, and who still on occasion invade my apartment in my dreams, once more invade my waking conscious mind, as they did in my youth. All those poisonous snakes still, in the deepest strata of my unconscious mind, once more block my path "home," to myself, to what I know.

But maybe I'm beginning to overcome them. I know *something.* A small, fresh awareness is budding in my head. This time it doesn't take me long to glimpse beyond the veneer. It is only the right action that eludes me.

I visit Mother for the first time late in the afternoon of her second day at Haven. The moment I enter her room, my hope strengthens. Her bed stands next to a large window. Sunlight pours over her as she sleeps, a flood of light by which to read. Her newspaper lies unopened on her stomach, her hands resting over it. But it's there, delivered whole, untouched by another patient, and within her reach. She'll get it here every day, and she'll have plenty of light to read by. I lean over and kiss her. "Mother?"

She wakes, more or less.

We chat. Or, I chat. She half-listens and, periodically, she listens with her full attention, propped up by moments of her old energy. I tell her what's in the news. "Oh, isn't that fascinating!" I detail the election, the dispute over the Florida ballots. "Oh," she says, "I feel terrible that I didn't vote!"

I blanch, suddenly heartsick. Why did I so cavalierly toss away her ballot without a word? Voting was almost as much a part of her as driving. Working up another lie, I say, "I'm sorry. I must have accidentally put it with the junk mail."

"Oh, that's all right, honey. You can't do everything. You're doing just fine. I don't know what I'd do without you."

The nurse arrives with Mother's dinner and raises her bed. The nurse picks up a spoon, dips it into the mashed potatoes and places the spoon in Mother's mouth, which opens with childlike obedience. I watch, shock once more stunning me into silence, my heart small and helpless in its grasp. Mother opens her mouth like an infant while the nurse inserts the spoonful of food. One spoonful then another. Then that's it. Finished, Mother makes a rejecting sound, pushes the spoon aside and lies back down, closing her eyes.

Is this how my mother eats now? *What's going on here?* In *one day* my mother has suddenly become too weak to feed herself and doesn't even notice? The nurse lowers Mother's bed and leaves. Before I get past that shock, Mother's white hospital gown slips a little off her shoulder. I gape at her shoulder. Her skin is unnaturally shiny as her muscle-skeleton moves beneath it, slipping around, the skin loose over her stark anatomy, the two separate, skin and bone, no longer of a whole; no muscle. I can't hold back my tears. “I’m sorry, I’m sorry!” I haven’t seen her enough. I’ve made terrible mistakes. She’s so thin and weak!

“Don’t be sorry. You have nothing to be sorry for. I don’t know what I’d do without you. You’re doing everything you can.” But that’s her last lively moment for the day. After that she lies with her eyes half-closed. I weep as I leave her, crying all the way home and half the night.

What’s happened to my mother at Haven?

A song lyric, or chorus, answers at the back of my mind, *Slip-slipping away.*

Another Change

I cry for hours after my next few visits. Tears flood from my eyes the instant I leave her room. Finally I can't stand it any longer. I choose the perpetual ache of unshed tears behind my eyes and swelling in my throat to the tsunami of tears that flow on and off half the night in wrenching sobs that exhaust me, physically as well as emotionally. I can't keep doing that. I need all my strength to keep calling her, seeing her, fighting for her. Or so I tell myself, although for the most part, the reality is that I no longer have to fight for her pain medication. She gets more than enough. At the moment I fight this hospital only to get her the salads she still wants. When I tell her I'm ready to give up that fight, she implores, "Oh, don't stop fighting!" So I don't. I shut off further crying. I'll cry when she's dead.

Which might be sooner rather than later.

I've only spoken to her new physician, Dr. Woo, on the phone. He seemed all right until, two weeks in, the pharmacy called to tell me that Woo's latest antibiotic prescription for Mother is a drug to which she is allergic. I thanked the pharmacist for being so alert. Then I called Woo to ask how he'd missed her allergy. He said, "I didn't have her chart in front of me."

***

As before, most of my visits are short and late in the day. I gave up my apartment hunt a month ago when Scary Ron was evicted (for not paying his rent, rather than for flipping lit cigarette butts on the grass right next to the apartment building). But I still wake every hour. After four awakenings I still spend the rest of the night staring at the inside of my eyelids and then take all day to drag myself out of bed. Exhaustion aches in my veins. My blood crawls along. I'm certain I've sustained heart damage from the noise and hostility of my "home." My immune system is still lagging. I still have to get to Cedars for my shots.

On the days I do visit Mother, I can hardly move to pull on my clothes and chase the two consecutive buses (half the time I am dizzy and short of breath after that run). I have to get to Haven early enough to get home before dusk, a vital time frame because of the long walk from the bus stop to my apartment. Last year a crazy guy was lurking in the bushes en route; he followed me to my apartment. Three years before, a man was found in his carjacked vehicle parked across the street from my apartment with his throat slit. I'm desperate to get home before dark.

But Mother suffers constantly from my desperation and desertion, especially since I speak with her less and less on the phone: she sleeps most of the time. They must drug her more heavily here than at any other facility. Should I confront them about overmedicating her? But the drugs keep her pain from returning—and, I have to admit, her insane calls to me have stopped. But then she needs me to come more often, and earlier, so I can stay later. But no matter how hard I try, I just can't seem to do it.

I wonder, *But wouldn't she do it for me?*

***

When I do finally arrive, Mother's half-deaf roommate, a woman with slurred speech, is blasting the overhead wall television. That torturous sound pounds into and merges with the emotional pain I feel at seeing Mother a little more frail and lost with each visit.

At first we have small conversations. I continue to give her election updates, Bush, Gore, Florida, the historic moment, the melodrama from hell—Bush just *can't* be the next president!—the most interesting thing I can divulge. In the beginning I see her old energy and fascination. "Oh, isn't that interesting," she says. But over the days and weeks, our conversations contract. She speaks less and less, instead staring into the distance.

Then the tone of her responses dims.

How has this happened so fast?

When she first came to Haven she'd exclaimed, with energy and mental fluency, "Oh, I feel terrible that I didn't vote!" Now only one month later her exclamations have shrunk to mere habit, her interest remembered, weakly mimicked, not felt. "How interesting!" Her fascination an apparition, a mirage. My mirage, the one I want to believe.

She has her own, less attractive. She sometimes drifts in her somnolent state into hallucinations. "I just came back from a concert. I tried to call you. Where were you?" "Put my shoes on, honey. I have to go out. I have to go to the doctor... Maybe you better take off my shoes. I don't think I can go out."

But each day her delusions darken more, transmogrifying her lifelong fears of getting lost into nightmarish scenarios of being alone, imperiled and terrified. "My car is broken down and I'm in Canada but I don't know where. I don't know anyone here. How will I get home?" "I'm in my office downtown. No one else is here. I'm afraid!" "Help me! I'm in Las Vegas! Someone stole my purse. I have no money. I can't call anyone. I can't get home! Help me! Help me!" Then she is again in Mexico, shouting, "Policia! Policia!" Her hallucinations are all fraught with fear, and unless I'm there, she eventually screams for help.

One nurse comforts her by holding her hand for five minutes. But I've come to realize the other nurses ignore her initial agitation and muttering as well as all her new symptoms—those that have erupted in Haven along with her multiplying hallucinations: a restless, anguished tossing and twitching and talking to herself loudly with panicky little gestures. When she starts screaming, the other nurses silence her by giving her more drugs. She sleeps more and more. She is going downhill so fast I can't keep up.

But she isn't in physical pain.

But her pressure sore will never heal.

I see this now. She's too weak, too thin, too drugged, too infected. She's still got the catheter, which keeps causing urethral or intrauterine infections; I can't get it clear. What I do understand is that she's got two infections right now for which she takes three antibiotics, and she's bound to hit an infection that can only be stopped by a drug to which she's allergic. She's allergic to sulfa drugs, the penicillin family and another class of drugs, one member of which being the drug Woo had negligently prescribed. She's emaciated and—forget bed exercises. She probably wouldn't even understand the concept now. "Move or die." George, the physical therapist at Meadows, wasn't lying about that.

One morning I wake to find six messages on my answering machine. My stomach lurches, my heart clenches. I can barely remember when I used to be glad to see that someone had called me. These messages come from Grace, Sid Lucy and the Haven nurses. Mother is at Cedars. "She wasn't answering us," the Haven nurse tells me when I call. "We yelled at her but she wasn't waking up. Pretty soon she wouldn't be breathing."

Frantic at what Mother must be going through, I throw on some clothes and call a cab. At the Cedars ER, I locate Mother in a small room. An oxygen tube projects from her nose. She's awake. I kiss her cheeks and stroke her face over and over, gently. She seems to relax a little.

"How are you doing?" I ask.

"I've felt better." That's what she always used to say when she had a flu and it was finally terrible enough to send her grudgingly to the doctor.

I go back into the ER. A nurse points Mother's doctor out to me. A tallish man in his mid-forties with gray hair and beard, wearing hospital blues, he stands leaning over a counter writing up what looks like a chart. I introduce myself and ask about my mother.

"She's dehydrated and she has pneumonia."

I'm not surprised but I feel my last corpuscle of credulity shrivel. Despite everything, I've raced down one of

Mother's corridors of denial. *Oh, I just can't believe it!* I've become disillusioned about Haven, but still the administrator's encouraging promise about patients recovering from pressure sores has remained with me to some degree. But once more she hasn't even received basic care. I say, "Aren't *any* of these places any good?"

The doctor pauses before answering. He reflects. "In my experience, no."

I stare at him. Of course this truth is not news, yet it wipes me out. *How is it possible, in this century, in this country?* Once more I've believed an image, rather than what I know to be true.

I start to turn away. Then I recall something and turn back. "Her HMO doctor saw her yesterday." It was the one visit per month, or per two months, by Dr. Woo, whom I still haven't met (and never will). The Cedars doctor pauses in his writing and looks back at me. Our eyes meet. He raises his brows in disgust, cynicism, sorrow and regret. We hold each other's eyes a moment. Then he turns back to the paper he's writing on.

Last time the good Dr. Woo missed Mother's drug allergy because he didn't bother to put her chart in front of him. This time he'd had her body and still missed everything.

Yet I miss things, too. Between the stress of my apartment and trying to save Mother, I'm falling apart more each day, just like she is. I cannot think straight. My actions make no sense. She'll never get back her mind or walk again. She'll never heal from the pressure sore. She'll never go home or anywhere else. Mother once told me that she wouldn't mind living in a nursing home if she could have her tapes and books. But now, with finality, I realize that was never a possibility. Not even before she forgot how to work a portable radio.

No books or tapes for Mother. If such places exist, they're well beyond our income scale. In any case today she would no longer recognize their value anyway.

For her sake, I want her to die. So do Grace, Sid and Lucy. Grace, Sid and I have begun to talk about it in our nightly conversations. We want her suffering to end. But despite our conversations and prayers for her death, I find myself fighting for her life.

Or do I just fight the dragon? I refuse to accept that the dragon always wins. But this is the battle that counts for *us* and we've already lost. That is what I refuse to accept, until, as rapidly as everything else at Haven, refusal becomes impossible.

Woo

Cedars sends Mother back to Haven later that afternoon. The next day I talk to Woo on the phone. I address Mother's dehydration and pneumonia. Woo responds, "When a patient has pneumonia," he relates, "the cough has a particular sound. I didn't hear it."

I resist the urge to tell him to get his hearing fixed. I think that I'll need his help as long as he's Mother's doctor. "My mother's breath is very short. I'm concerned she doesn't get enough oxygen."

"They can test her every day."

Well, that's interesting. "Can you arrange it? Would you write that down as an order?" Ryan always had to write down his orders, for those nurses who would read them.

When Woo agrees, I ask about the dehydration.

"It's hard to tell if a patient is dehydrated." He adds, "Dehydration is a major problem at these hospitals. But there's a blood test she can get every Monday."

Well, I think, then it's not that hard. And if dehydration is a major problem at these hospitals, why not run the test routinely? "Will you order that for her, too, please, and write it for the nurses?"

A small chuckle. "So you see how things work there."

"Yes, I do." Barely better than at Meadows. *And I see how you work, too,* although of course I don't say this, either. "Her eyes always have this thick film over them."

"It wasn't there when I came."

Should he also get his eyes fixed? Well, he saw her in the morning. I'm always there in the afternoon. Mother's friend Robbie, who comes in the evening for a few minutes after work, also sees the cloudy film. But maybe it isn't there in the morning. I don't really believe this but I drop the subject. Mother isn't up for a cataract operation anyway, if that's the cause.

Indeed, she isn't up for Haven. Next time I visit I find her lying on her back. I address the nurse helping the other patient. "My mother's supposed to be on her side and turned every two hours." That much I've finally learned.

"We'll be bringing in her dinner pretty soon."

That sounds reasonable but less so as forty-five minutes pass, there's no food and still no one has turned her. I complain to the charge nurse when I leave but I don't have the strength to stay and make sure she does it.

I continue resisting the urge to weep. I don't know how I hold back the tears. Day after day, Mother's newspaper, unread, remains beneath her folded hands, half off her stomach. Though bathed in sunlight, she's never opened the paper once since she's come to Haven. Finally, I say, "Do you think I should stop the paper for a while?" I want her to say no, if not with her old unyielding iron will then at least with a hint of vigor. Her paper! The paper she read every day of her adult life, cover to cover, that became on this journey her lifeline to the world outside, and that she begged for only weeks ago at Meadows.

"I don't know. I guess so."

The next day I cancel her subscription. I think about how she looks and behaves, her medical condition, the people taking care of her. I think about how she measured quality of life, how much of it was her mind. I think that the only thing keeping her alive now is that the fight she's fought all her life has become a cellular habit. Her body just won't let go. "She has a strong heart," Grace says when we talk about praying for her release from suffering. But even with that fight, that heart, even one more month of life is inconceivable. I call Woo and ask for the last, single thing that might comfort her for however long she has left. I realize I've been sucking up to him for just such a favor.

"I want to move her to hospice care." It's supposed to be better than hospital care. They specialize in making the patient comfortable through their last days. My fight has collapsed. I know that's where we are.

But Dr. Woo explains the rules. "To qualify for hospice care, your mother must have a specific terminal illness that gives her six months or less to live."

"Well, how long do you think she has?"

"Anywhere from two weeks to two years."

"Two years?" I gasp. What is he talking about? "She's starving. You said so yourself."

"That's not exactly what I said."

What he said, exactly, was that my mother has less than eighteen per cent of the protein necessary for life in her body. "It's the meaning of what you said. She's dying."

"You never know. She might rally."

Rally? Is he crazy? I'm floored. Staggered. Speechless. Falling over the bridge. I argue with him but he won't send her. I don't understand. Why not? Who would it hurt? But I don't know how to make it happen. I can't convince him.

Poor Mother. It's still just me, making you as comfortable as I can.

On the phone I ask Mother about her radio. The saga of the radio. "Oh, that little radio is saving my sanity!" she'd cried out, repeating her excited gratitude the moment I brought it to her after her operation and at every place to which she's gone since. Although she could never remember how to turn it on or off, she somehow worked her way through the knobs and buttons to get her classical music station with some frequency. During her second stay at Meadows, the portable radio fell through the bars of her bed and broke. I brought a plug-in and planted it on the small table behind her head. I set it for classical music loud enough for her to hear yet low enough to disturb no one else.

"But how can I reach it? How will I change the station?"

"You won't. That's how you lose your music. Then you don't find it again. Then the radio falls while you're fiddling with the dials. Or someone else moves the radio to make your bed and drops it. If I leave it on this table turned on all the time, you'll always hear it and no one else will have a reason to touch it."

She grumbled assent.

Then I would visit her and find it turned off. Someone had turned it off. Or I'd come in and a rock station would be blasting.

Here at Haven I don't find rock but still her radio is frequently off. Mother says now, "Oh, I don't know." Usually she is too drugged to reach the low morale she experienced at Meadows; she has too little awareness to become depressed by her new "caretakers." But losing her music brings back the despair. "The volume is too low. I can't hear it."

The next time I come in, I only hear Mother's roommate's blasting television. As always I try to ignore it and suppress the pain it creates in my head and the frenzy to get away. I pay attention to Mother, today, to her radio. It is silent. I check and find it broken.

What happened to her radio? How can they be so insensitive, here, too? Does no one anywhere see my mother as anything more than another interchangeable old woman who is dying? I think again about hospice care. Would they have kept her classical music on, to give her peace and joy? In a loving environment would her hallucinations have been kinder? Why couldn't Woo have helped?

I promise Mother I'll get her radio fixed or replaced. Her time is coming and I feel I'll somehow know when it happens. I'll come to her then and stay with her. I will hold her hand as she goes, and the last sound she hears will be her classical music playing from the radio, escorting her out.

I've seen one sentimental movie too many.

"I'll bring a new radio next time."

"It's really essential," she asserts. This would once have been a command. But now she speaks vaguely. The words rising on her shallow breath are only an echo of her old, stubborn, emphatic, vital self. Her literary self. *It's really essential.* These words belong to the ghost of a woman who loved classical music, who has voiced her last wish. The words arise from the last spark of the spirit that is she. But I'm unable to get to a store to buy a new radio before my next visit.

Last Appearance

I sit by her bed in Haven, the third hospital, and fourth and last stop on her dreadful journey, not even six months after her surgery. I hold her hand that is now always cold. She lies today a little on her side. Through her half-closed, film-clouded eyes she gazes in silence, as she has come to do, into an unfathomable distance. She gazes without looking, no longer curious, her spirit subdued, her animation quiescent. When she does speak, there is no vitality; and her curiosity about politics and health care and everything else is gone, along with her jokes, puns and the smile that changed over a lifetime. She who always had questions, exclamations, insights and that great laughter seems only to rest in a kind of waiting state, like a crow I once saw that had been run over. Its black eyes glazed, it stood patiently on the grass, tottering a little, looking at me as it waited to die.

Every once in a while Mother gives my hand a little squeeze. *I still know you. I still love you. I know you're here.*

But for how much longer?

I squeeze back. But I've watched her memories erased more each day by the medical system, its experts with their apathy, their food devoid of nutrition, their drugs. Their lack of humanity. They've eradicated her past and stolen her future.

"Do you still see the people we used to know?" she asks me from the distant place she now inhabits. This is her old warmth toward others, her love of her friends and curiosity about their lives, but without her old passion. Another ghost. The people we used to know. The people I called and to whom I said, "If you want to talk to my mother while she still remembers you, now's the time."

Roger says, "I'm glad I saw her while she was still herself." But in some cases I was too late, or they were. "The people we used to know" are her dear friends of decades, sometimes of more than half-a-century, to whom she now speaks politely. "I don't think she knew who I was," say Alta, Anna, Carmella, Mari.

"Yes," I tell Mother softly, "I still see them."

After a moment I rise and lean over her, speaking close to her ear, intimately, privately. "Close your eyes. Let's do a meditation." Perhaps I can bring a touch of joy into this terrible place to which she has come.

Her eyes close and she seems to listen as I say softly, "Remember when you were young, how you loved the surf. Imagine yourself on the water again, the salt foam all about you, remember and feel it again, how you bodysurfed to the shore. Feel it again, the joy, the beach. Feel the sun on your back, and how you flew in to shore on the waves. Let yourself feel the joy, the sun, the water swooshing over you."

I finish. Her eyes open. She looks at me with innocence and says in a childlike voice, "Now?"

I sink back into my chair. "Yes. Now." But I know she doesn't understand and I haven't the heart to repeat it for her. She doesn't ask for a repetition. It's already gone. She's forgotten I said anything at all. Silence falls over us. As her mind travels through drug-imposed vagaries, mine also drifts. Everything Mother saw and did in her life is ceasing to be part of her even before she dies. How soon before she forgets the last piece of her history, the last person in her life?

I sit here beside her, holding her hand that I cannot make warm, and I think about everything that formed her personality—her love of learning, the knowledge about health she gained and joyfully shared with others, all the joy she's known, her second marriage and great love, our estrangement and loving reconciliation. I think about the massive shifts in our relationship. I think that if she no longer knows me, if she forgets who I am as she's forgotten her friends, if all her experiences and loving relationships are obliterated and, with them, her identity, then what has any of it mattered?

Periodically, she squeezes my hand or I, hers, and I think about my own life, my smile that I so hated when I was young, my efforts to find my "true self," to write, to get well; my friends; my own successes and mistakes; and how profoundly my mother's and my relationship changed and changed me: what was it all for? I cannot bear the silence and speak into it.

"I might be getting another apartment." At best I expect an amorphous nod. But she raises her head a little off the pillow. She looks at me, her eyes lighting up with life and lucidity. "No kidding!" A familiar exclamation; a return to herself. "How did it happen?" Eyes bright with her old vigor and intelligence, from the days when we shared our lives with each other.

I tell her how I found the place when I started looking eight months before and have kept in touch with the owner. "I never thought I'd get it—a one-bedroom for five hundred—a miracle—a tenant is leaving—"

But she is already lying back.

I keep talking, narrating. Even though the light has faded from her face and I know it is useless, I tell her. "And I'm first on the list…"

I stop. Her eyes gaze once more into that horizon from which there is no return. This has been her last appearance, for love, reaching out for a final, shared, cherished experience with me.

I look at her pale face, the little open mouth, and her hair thin and white; at her clouded, half-closed eyes and her expression of patient waiting, for death. I remember when her deteriorating mind reminded me of sand castles washed away by the tide. Now as I sit here, her mind seems to me to slip beneath her illness like ancient deserted cities overgrown with furious green jungle; her inquisitive mind and brilliance vanishing like the old, once fabulous civilizations buried beneath desert dust; like all the places of the past that once so fascinated her.

The next time I come to see her, I find none of her treasures on her bed.

Lost Treasures

I return without the new radio I promised to obtain. I haven't been able to get to a store. As I approach her, I see her purse, black bag and huge hardback herb book sitting on the shelf across the room from her bed. Why isn't she upset, weeping, angrily demanding them? I strive for a casual tone. "Don't you want these on your bed?" I bring over her purse and the big herb book. As I plant them beside her, where she can reach them, she pushes at them ineffectually with tremulous fingers and gestures toward the shelf. "You better put them back, dear," she declares, courteously. "Someone will want them."

"They're yours." I squeeze her hand.

She squeezes back, a gesture. "You better put them back, dear," she repeats, her tone expressing consideration for whoever owns them.

I return them to the shelf. I know what this means. Answered prayers. But my whole self is not in them. I don't want to lose her. In fact with another part of my mind I still somehow expect—not that she can recover; I do not articulate to myself the word "recovery"—but that she won't die. That I'm wrong about her condition. About what I see with my own eyes.

She'll come back as she always has. She will find clemency in life, not death. Her laughter will return as it always has. Her history holds her on this world and laughter is not only hers but ours, an ineradicable bond in our second relationship. She has to come back. To "rally."

But at the same time I know her luck is gone. As I leave her room today, her nurse mentions, "Your mother's developing another small pressure sore on her back."

Devastated but not surprised, I nod. But I know she won't live long enough for it to become another agonizing wound. She's already been killed by the first one.

Last Visit

A week later, passing Mother's roommate, I try as usual to ignore the woman's television blasting overhead from the wall. But this time I'm so weary and nerve-wracked that I cringe. If possible I sleep even less and have even less energy to make food, so I rarely eat. (I've lost fifteen pounds and am delightfully slender again, as I was at sixteen, just before the big bulge, I cannot help but note in erratic, self-centered moments.) I lie down between any slightest effort. Just breathing seems to require every thread of energy I can stitch together; and then I run for the first bus, panting, then the second, as I will run when I leave here to get home before dark.

If I get the other apartment, I'll have a home base from which to help my mother. It will be quiet and I will sleep. If I don't get it, I won't survive, either.

As I approach Mother's bed, she stares at me. "Alexa?" Incredulous, afraid to hope. "Is it you?"

"Yes." I gently take her hand and kiss her cheek. "I'm here."

"I thought you were dead! I was going to kill myself!"

"No, it's all right. I'm all right. I'm here."

I sit and keep her hand in mine. She clings tightly to it and then begins to relax. I no longer attempt to fill the silence. She has nothing more to say, ask, opine. She just wants me with her. She wants the warm animal comfort of my presence, the human comfort of sharing the end of her life with me, her daughter, in love.

But today is different, unnerving. In the last several days her twitching and trembling has worsened. Now, once assured that I haven't died, that I'm really alive and with her, she rocks herself in a weird, obsessive way. Lost in a field of pharmaceutical dreams and side effects, she rocks forward and back, forward and back in her bed.

It is agony to watch her. She reminds me of an inmate in The Snake Pit, a madhouse of the past and another literary reference Mother and I once shared; a reference she would no longer recognize should I mention it to her.

The nurse stops by to tell me, "She took off her gown this morning." She giggles. "We have trouble getting her to keep it on."

I too have trouble. Mother keeps pulling it down. I lean over and keep pulling it back up over her fragile, wasted shoulders. "Aren't you cold?"

"Yes."

"Then you need to keep this gown over you. And the blankets."

She nods then pushes the gown down again, shoving the blankets away from her chest, as if shedding her flesh, trying to push away anything that might keep her on this plane. I pull them back over her. She leaves them alone for a while.

I sit next to her. The blasting television makes me yearn to weep or break free of a nonexistent straight jacket. My fear of getting home in the dark grows more each day, and through the wide window I see the sun fading to that pitch of light that means if I don't leave right this second, I won't make it.

Sometimes I stay only twenty minutes, more rarely an hour. But it's never enough time, not remotely, and again today I've gotten here too late to give her even that hour, indeed, no more than half that. After I rise to leave. I say what I always say. "I need to leave now to beat the dark. The cab is so expensive."

Mother never wants me to go, but whenever I tell her it's getting dark and I have very little cab money, her old fear of not having money resurfaces dimly. She responds, lonely and sad, "Oh. All right. I guess so." But now she clutches my hand. "Don't go! I don't want you to go yet!" My mother has never clutched my hand and begged me to stay longer. "Please don't go," she implores me.

Compelled, I hold her hand. Besides me, only Robbie comes here; she works close enough to Haven to visit Mother many evenings. But she can stay for even shorter visits. And how much do these visits help Mother? She used to know when I was absent. "When are you coming? When will you be back?" She knew when I didn't come. She missed me being there with a desperate grief that will forever clench my heart as her hand clenches mine in this moment. But when Robbie comes in the evenings or I visit Mother in the afternoon, she's forgotten minutes later. For her it's as if no one has come.

But I sit down again, dismissing the oncoming dark. Mother lies back and, holding my hand, resumes her strange rocking. I have to stay. But every cell in my body feels beaten up, and Mother's roommate's ear-splitting television drives the breath from my body. It shreds my brain worse than the TV at my apartment coming through the ceiling because this one is *right here.* I have to stay.

But I want go home, lie on my bed, shove my earplugs in up to my eyeballs; I have to reduce the blasting of the television, which is unbearable; and I have to eat. I'm starving—ravenous. I can't afford to eat out or order in; I refuse to eat foods that will make me sicker, so I lie in bed for hours until I gather enough strength to get up and make something healthy. But I yet to do that today. *I have to go! Don't you understand why?* But as these thoughts and sensations shutter through me, the deeper truth shifts into view.

Before her operation Mother signed her Durable Power of Attorney for Health Care over to me. In it she scrawled by hand, "I strongly desire constant relief from pain even if large amounts, etc., shorten my life. And all things to make me comfortable."

Are you comfortable, Mother, rocking away there? You're not in pain anymore. Oh, but Mother, you don't look yourself. I sit with you, our hands entwined. We signal each other with squeezes. But you rock and rock yourself, and I cannot help you at all.

With nothing in my veins but fatigue and hunger and nothing in my skull but this agonizing noise, I must, but cannot, process my breaking heart.

***

The truth is that I cannot stand to see you like this, rocking and rocking with that childlike expression in your clouded, half-closed eyes.

The truth is that I cannot bear to see your body emaciated and your newspaper gone and your treasures lying on the shelf across the room, unwanted, abandoned.

The truth is that I have to go outside into the fresh air beneath the last fading rays of the setting sun, away from the white room and lightless agony of watching you rock yourself to death.

The truth is that I have to get away from the pain of watching my mother leave me and of my having to wish her well on her departure.

I hold on for another twenty minutes then call a cab. As I rise to leave, Mother cries out, "Oh, can't you stay longer?" These are her only words in the last twenty minutes, the only energy she has shown.

I apologize. I embrace her. She coughs, her deep chesty cough. She still has pneumonia. I jump back. Woo says she's not contagious but he's not the epitome of medical accuracy.

I can't stay. I just can't. *Forgive me.* "I'll be back soon."

Outside her room I start down the hall. It's harder than ever to suppress my tears but habit saves me. Then behind me I hear Mother shouting, "John! John!" John who? John was Mitch's middle name. My father called himself Jon although his name was Matthew. Does Mother yell for her beloved husband? Her youth? Does the name John somehow graft her entire history back onto her mind? Her tone is demanding and frantic.

I stop at the nurses' station. "I don't want her to suffer," I instruct Reginald, her charge nurse tonight, a tallish Filipino man in his early thirties. "Don't wait till she starts yelling before you give her a sedative. Give her the pill the minute you see she's agitated."

He objects. "If we give her too many sedatives, she becomes non-responsive." "Non-responsive." Now part of my vocabulary. Reginald means that she will first not wake and then not breathe. That was the concern that impelled them to send Mother to Cedars. Too many drugs then. But now too few.

"Give it to her," I say flatly. "If you think there's a legal problem, call the doctor. Ask him to call me. I'll agree to what he says." I hope he won't object. Mother's hallucinations torment her as much as the nurses and CNAs used to do, would do now, were she more aware. She wanted to be kept comfortable. I will keep her comfortable. "She never wanted to be like this." I look Reginald in the eyes. "Would you?"

His eyes widen just a little. Recognition crystallizes in them. No. He wouldn't.

"Give her the sedatives. If she dies, she dies."

Dr. Woo never calls me. I guess it's not a problem.

The Call

I'm a wreck as I sit on the stoop in front of Haven. Waiting in the night for the cab, I promise Mother and myself that I'll do better next time. I'll bring my earplugs; why haven't I thought of that before? That will cut the worst edge off the TV volume. And I'll come earlier. And more often. Somehow, I'll do it. I will, as Mother would phrase it, "turn over a new leaf." Today is the last Thursday in December. Monday is New Year's. I swear I'll go Sunday and Monday, too. And bring her a radio. I'll make it up to her.

But on this century-ending holiday weekend, the horrible people leave my apartment building. The building manager, my upstairs neighbor, the latest rock musician down the hall: they leave the city. Sunday I sit on the porch and it is quiet. No one passes me, nukes me with a glance of hatred. It's as if an evil spell has lifted off the building, and I sit here, knees up, back to the porch wall, in the quiet, in a stupor, as if pinned. Even as I command myself to go see Mother, the very thought of the bus and the television in Mother's room sets my hackles rising.

And then, again, the truth: What will Mother be like? Will she be rocking again? Will she have forgotten me?

I just sit on the porch and stare at the tree across the street and inhale its goodness.

Monday passes the same way. I go inside at 5:30 and call Mother. There's no answer. I call Reginald. "She's sleeping," he says.

"How is she?"

He says, "She's better today. She's eating more. She kept asking for more food."

I picture Mother, the bed raised to support her in a sitting position as her little mouth opens, her eyes wide and childlike, as Reginald offers her a spoonful of food. "Ahhh!

Ahhh!" More! More! I wonder, Is this her old will to live reasserting itself? Her cellular habit of fighting poverty and her fear of poverty, conquering cancer, surviving her grief at losing Mitch, the love of her life, and then fighting Alzheimer's—beginning to "lick it": Is she fighting again, suddenly, for life?

Grace, Sidney, Lucy and me, we all hope and pray for my mother's misery to end.

She's better today.

I go back outside to sit on the apartment porch. The warm Los Angeles December night brushes my face. I think, *Oh, god. Don't rally. Don't rally.* After a while I go back inside and lie down. I'll try her later. Maybe she'll be awake and we can talk. I will definitely see her tomorrow. Then I'll get her radio fixed or replaced.

At ten the phone rings. It's Reginald. "Alexa?" he verifies.

"Yes."

There is a pause. Then he says, "Your mother's passed. We checked on her at 9:30. She was sleeping..."

I'm aware of holding onto the phone. My mouth seems unable to catch onto words. My voice won't produce any sounds that might cohere. She clung to me, and begged me to stay, and that was the last time I saw her alive.

I'd said to Reginald, "Give her the sedative. If she dies, she dies." And so she did.

I manage a few words. "I'll be right there." But I sit back on my bed. My brain cells stumble around in disorder. It takes me almost an hour to call Sid and Grace (we decide not to wake Lucy; I'll call her in the morning), figure out what to wear, put it on and call a cab.

I kept leaving her early to save cab money. For what? Emergencies. I've been crazy! *This* is not the emergency. Her life was the emergency, not her death. What's wrong with me?

Her room is silent for once, the television off. It's after eleven. Her roommate greets me. She knows what has happened. "She was okay this afternoon. I'm sorry."

I thank her and continue to my mother. I close the curtain around the bed where Mother lies covered by a sheet, and pull back the sheet. Mother lies on her back in her white hospital gown. She looks alive.

Her arms are crossed over her chest. Her mouth is slightly parted, as if she's only paused, mid-breath, mid-sentence, suspended in time. Her lids are half-closed over her film-clouded brown eyes through which she still seems to gaze with that look of patient waiting, of slow leaving, now with a vague puzzlement at what has happened to her after a good life, a constant fight, another victory on the horizon.

I can't stand to see this.

No matter how she looks, I have to remind myself, *she's dead.*

I suppress the urge to regurgitate. I'm not aware of any smell in the room, but perhaps you don't need to literally smell death to know its presence.

I try to close her mouth, pushing up on her lower jaw. I'm not sure why I do this—some vague notion of "dignity in death," a primordial human urge, or maybe it's just something I got from movies and television shows. In any case it doesn't work. Her skin is still warm and pliant but her jaw moves only a little and only so long as I keep pressure on it. The moment I let go, her jaw drops back where it was. I move it up a fraction of an inch, it moves back down. It won't hold the slightest readjustment.

I try to close her eyelids but they too stay fixed, the skin still warm and soft, and fragile.

"Please let me close your eyes," I beg her quietly.

But she is being her old, stubborn self.

My tears spill out. I can't reconcile her looking alive and being dead; the stubbornness of her jaw to close; the refusal of her lids to shut over the clouded eyes gazing into nothing, yet looking as if her magnificent imagination might linger still; as if her once extraordinary intelligence still rested behind those eyes.

I hadn't thought she'd make it through the year but she's surprised me. Her will to live carried her into the first night of the new year of the new century.

I pull the sheet back over her and cross the room to the shelf. I run my hands over her purse, her ratty black bag, some books people have brought her that I never noticed before. I pick up a card and see it was sent to her and signed by her whole exercise class, which she attended almost until the operation. I put it down again, next to the broken radio, neatly wrapped in its cord. I will take all this home tonight. I pick up her beloved herb book and open it. There on the inside leaf my phone number is scribbled at all angles into every square inch.

I lay the book back down and return to her bed. I have to see her again. I pull the sheet back. She still looks alive.

One of her first hallucinations occurred a few months ago. That night on the phone, when I called to find out how my mother was, her nurse told me, "When I went into her room, she was holding her phone and talking to the receiver, 'Mother! Mother!' I asked her if she was talking to herself and she said, 'Yes.'" Hearing this, I'd hung up, weeping. But now I understand my mother was not quite as demented as I thought. I touch her cold hand, no colder than it has been during the last months, with her gold wedding band on it. I think, *She never forgot Mitch or me. She remembered the love at the core of her personality and life to the last.* Her luck held after all. Then I speak quietly, so that her roommate won't hear me.

"Mother! Mother! Mother!"

Book Six

The Speed of Light

March, 2001

DHS

Tears press at my eyes and wet my lashes. A few droplets escape down my face. It's not really that I never cry but that I haven't let go with the wracking sobs that I know demand release.

The month after Mother died, Annette, the Department of Health Services investigator, called me on a Saturday morning. Her grandchildren playing noisily in the background, she apologized for bothering me on the weekend.

"Oh, no," I said, "I can't tell you how much I appreciate you taking your personal time to call me. What did you find out?"

Annette said, "The home health care nurses who saw your mother at the residential care facility, Oasis, missed your mother's dehydration and impacted bowel. Also, they were supposed to re-evaluate her every three days. They only did it once in the two weeks she was there."

Not entirely surprised by any new revelation, still I felt sick with this news. They really did abandon her. "What about the ER?"

"The nurses at your mother's ER cleaned and bandaged one of her legs. But they didn't examine the other one, even though both legs were bandaged. The nurses' notes don't say anything about a pressure sore on her back."

"How could they not say anything? When they cleaned out her impacted bowel, they'd have been looking right at it."

"We can't prove it was there at the time."

"But Dr. Ryan told me it was a Stage IV when she got to Orchards, and Orchards is just blocks from the ER." Orchards had called Ryan to report that wound the moment they examined Mother and discovered it. Orchards even took pictures. I said, "Maybe the ER didn't say anything about the pressure sore because they caused it."

"We can't prove that," Annette repeats with compassion.

But my mind keeps unwinding. Mother's skin was so fragile! A pressure sore results from not turning a patient, not examining their skin. My mother was in the ER for thirty-six hours on those hard beds with nurses who couldn't even be bothered to clean and re-bandage the obvious wound on her leg. They must not have turned her, either, or examined her skin. What Annette told me just confirmed what I'd thought before. *The ER gave her the pressure sore. The ER killed my mother.* "And Meadows?"

"We can't do anything about Meadows missing your mother's pneumonia. However, the law says that all accusations of abuse must be reported to the hospital administrator, who must pass them on to us. The administrator never reported anything to us. We're citing them for Rory's abuse and for not reporting it. They're denying you ever complained about Georgia. But their records show she was removed from your mother's room, so we're able to cite them for abuse on that, too."

I thanked her. We hung up. I went back to bed for the rest of the day and lay staring at the ceiling.

I never complained about Orchards; she was only there four awful days and I didn't really know the situation. I didn't have anything specific about Haven; their lousy care seemed standard; maybe I was wrong. And I hadn't yet complained about Oasis. I had to believe that there was one place on Mother's journey, one group of people, who were kind to her. Who took care of her. In her last month Mother no longer remembered Rose or her assistants, whom she had loved more than she had distrusted. But I reminded her, "You walked up and down their driveway every day."

"Oh, yes," Mother said, her tone distant. "I remember that."

But a few weeks ago Camilla changed my mind. Camilla said, "They should never have accepted your mother with a bedsore."

"Why not?"

"Any open pressure sore requires skilled nursing care because any open pressure sore can become infected and life-threatening."

"But Oasis is a non-nursing board and care. It's only residential. They told me from the start."

"Then they shouldn't have taken your mother with a pressure sore. That was their first mistake," Camilla continued. "Once the sore reached the stage that it needed to be cleaned and bandaged, Rose should have known she was in over her head. She should immediately have contacted you and let you know your mother had to be returned to skilled nursing care."

These words pitched me deeper yet into the midnight mind-numbing grief already holding me enthrall.

Camilla added, "You can't develop a Stage IV Pressure Sore in thirty-six hours. It couldn't have happened at the ER. It had to have happened before then."

And, indeed, further investigation has exposed Rose's lies. Mother's pressure sore must have gone to Stage IV at Oasis. At any rate, the medical records show that my mother deteriorated more severely during her two weeks there than anywhere else.

Fear

Beneath the overcast gloom I stare at the broken cement path before me. Through my blurred gaze I conjure a picture of a distant past. The walkway is transformed into a clean, flat white. On either side of it there rise slender green stems bent by the tomatoes growing on them, that Mother planted. The bright red fruit of my childhood.

Through the years other inhabitants arrived uninvited. Wasps once built a nest into the outer wall of the living room (happily, I never saw them); and mice came briefly but in memorable force. Today ceiling rats are the latest unwelcome dwellers of my mother's house. While I delay extermination, the industrious rodents continue to munch up one of the off-white ceiling panels, which crumbles like some kind of box-filler onto the coffee table beneath. And of course there are the termites in the supporting beams. But the lethargy of grief slows my actions when I am not petrified by fear.

I got the other apartment. But I still rarely sleep and when I do, alarm wakes me in the night. For the first few seconds, the dark of my new bedroom is total. I don't know where I am. I inhale flames of panic up my chest with every breath. I have to choke back a scream.

I remember my mother in her last months. "Do you know where you are?" I would ask her.

"Well, no, not exactly..."

And where is she now? Now I'm the one who doesn't know where my mother is. The mystery of death: she's disappeared off the planet!

Why could I not save her? Fear saturates my cells. I am nauseous with terror at my helplessness. And within that fear lies yet another: the selfish one. What if I break *my* hip or for some other reason end up in a nursing care hospital? What happened to her could happen to me and I would not have someone even as inadequate as myself to be my advocate.

But then I would not be like her. I would be like her roommate, the "patient who always screams," in pain, terror, loneliness and helplessness, totally abandoned to the uncaring caretakers.

It's enough to wake anyone screaming in the night; although sometimes I can barely suppress a cry of fright in the daytime.

And when my terror subsides, I fall back into leaden sorrow.

Two Queens

Sitting in the yard of my mother's house in the silent gray morning, I watch crazy thoughts chase each other through my mind. One of them is the memory of a strange thing I read in my twenties.

It was a theory: the first new form of any kind—a cat, any kind of system, behavior, emotion, relationship, and so on—creates a "morphic resonance." This is a kind of quantum vibration that exists throughout and beyond the space-time continuum: Once the new form exists, it has always existed; it becomes what physics would call a "non-local event," instantaneously and simultaneously existing forward and backward in time, and in all directions of space – everywhere and everywhen at once.

This non-local or universal vibration—this morphic resonance—makes it possible for the next same form (the next cat, the next same behavior or emotion or relationship) to come into existence. And that new individual instance of the form strengthens its quantum resonance; and then that stronger resonance makes it easier for the next expression of the same form (the next cat, etc.) to exist.

A parallel to that theory, of a universal resonance, belongs to depth psychology. It's called an archetype. Archetypes are universal patterns. The pattern can be one of behavior, emotion, relationship, situation and so on. Ancient myths portray archetypes as sundry lovely or monstrous creatures, heroes and heroines, various divinities. Their stories dramatize various universal relationships and experiences. Every archetype lives in everyone; and their stories dramatize ours.

We unconsciously identify with the different archetypes and live them out just as unconsciously. Sometimes we can "individuate" away from them and into our individual experience of the archetype. But often individuals can become "possessed" by an archetype, unable to recognize where the universal pattern begins and one's individual experience ends.

Until we differentiate ourselves from the archetypes, their universal character usurps our individual identities.

Mother alternated between Nurturing Mother and the Devouring Mother; I played out the Rebellious Daughter and the Dutiful Daughter. Now a predominant archetype in my life is the God of Orphans. But there are others. One archetypal story that I'm living is the epic Sumerian myth I also read years ago.

This is the story:

Inanna, Goddess of the Upper World, Queen of Light, must visit her sister, Erishkigal. For Erishkigal, Dark Goddess of the Underworld, Queen of Darkness, is grieving. Erishkigal's husband has died and the Dark Goddess is in mourning.

Inanna, Goddess of the Upper World, personifies the universal experience of light, life, consciousness. Her sister, Erishkigal, Dark Goddess of the Underworld, personifies grief, death, the unconscious, the past.

Inanna knows her sister well. She wonders how, once in the Underworld, she will escape her sister's dark domain. And in fact when Inanna reaches the Underworld, Erishkigal takes a wooden stake and pins Inanna to the wall. And there she is, Inanna, Goddess of the Upper World, hanging in the Underworld, literally stuck in eternal darkness.

And that is my fear. I've suppressed so many tears they threaten to drown me if I dare release them, and the immobilizing darkness of all my buried memories presages a depression that will never end.

When I was eighteen and in that mental hospital, one of my fellow inmates, a woman a few years older than me, told me why she'd tried to commit suicide. "There was no me. There was just pain." I hadn't understood then, even though Rage at my mother—Rage, the archetype, the god—had equally possessed my own consciousness only weeks before. I too had lost my individuality to the universal pattern. But I never forgot her story, and now in the undertow of my despair, I understand.

I seek meaning in what happened to my mother. I struggle for transcendence, for light, for my own consciousness. This is why I've finally permitted back into my mind the full arc of my mother's and my half-century relationship, why I've allowed myself to relive it. But I've blundered. I have feared Erishkilgal, the power of the past, and I was right. Already my despondency is worse than it has been here. My reverie this morning has carried me deeper into the very depression I dread.

Until now, night has been the worst time. When I first lie down in the dark or wake to it in panic, my memories come as an onslaught. Grief possesses me. I fight for my own consciousness, my individual experience—myself. Now even in the daylight my small, personal, private grief becomes Grief, the divine possession, the universal pattern that traverses all time and space, the Grief that replaces my mother within me and then replaces us both.

The House

And now the house: Erishkigal, Goddess of the Dark, still demands my presence.

What to do with the two-bedroom, one-bath, deteriorated, Lilliputian house at the root of my mother's comfort and joy? Built in the teens around the time my mother herself was born, the house was conveyed from an unknown locality in 1946 to arrive on the lot where it now stands. At that time Los Angeles was so uncluttered you could tow whole parades of houses through the streets. Upon its arrival in Echo Park, Mother bought the house, lot and strip of land connecting both to the street with her last penny, for the retrospectively astounding price of thirty-nine hundred dollars.

The arcane, legal papers I've found clarify that when she divorced my father in 1947, the house, which she purchased "as a married woman," remained her sole possession.

Except at night in the bedroom of my new apartment, the interior of my mother's house is where I've felt most threatened by my banished memories and the desolation they can bring. The house, the past, the pain, the Underworld: until now I've managed to keep the worst of it at bay. But this morning that has changed. Yet I have no choice but to enter the house again.

I've come here with Susie three or four times for several hours each trip to clear out more of Mother's effects and treasures. I've also come with a contractor, three real estate agents and two estate sales people. And now I'm back with Susie.

I must fix the house, sell it or keep it. I must finish Mother's business and then get on with my own. The business of life. Even though her death, *that* death, it sometimes seems to me (as I hang nailed to Erishkigal's wall), makes all of Mother's victories irrelevant and causes me to wonder about the value of anything I or any of us does.

Titanic

I was born the same month and year that the first atom bombs fell. Under Mother's tutelage in my childhood and teens, I walked on peace marches with hundreds of thousands of Americans to "ban the bomb" and prevent nuclear war. And still, every year on August 6, Hiroshima survivors warn us about their experience. *I was knocked to the ground. I couldn't get up. I lifted my head and looked around. Everything was changed. Many people weren't getting up. Everyone was burned black. Their skin was hanging off them. I was—my face—was black. My parents didn't recognize me. I was thirteen. It was like hell. It was hell.*

The survivors speak. But Clinton never mentioned that accidental nuclear annihilation between the US and Russia is more possible than ever. Today, in the first year of the new century, almost ten years after the Cold War ended, the US and Russia still aim thousands of nuclear missiles at each other. Both sides are still on hair-trigger alert. Each president has *five minutes* to decide whether a radar blip is a bird, a weather balloon or a pre-emptive strike by the other side, and whether to launch their own weapons of thermonuclear war. The Russian early warning system barely functions. A few years ago Yeltsin didn't get the message about the launch of a Norwegian weather missile and literally came within ten seconds of retaliating against America for an imaginary attack. The world avoided thermonuclear war by ten seconds. And *still* both countries remain on hair-trigger alert, even as nuclear materials remain accessible to terrorists and nuclear weapons proliferate among nations.

Then what difference have I and the other seekers of peace made in the end? Do ancient goddesses and gods hopelessly compel us as they do humanity in the old tales?

Holding weapons of mass destruction, unwilling to give them up and indeed driven ever further toward wielding them at one another, we seem possessed by the Gods of Destruction. As if nuclear war were not enough, global warming threatens us with annihilation. Do universal patterns of emotion and behavior, which transcend our individual selves and our personal will, command our fate?

From parents who abuse their children to the adult children of those parents; from uncaring caretakers of the elderly to abusive world leaders and even whole populations that go mad: are we all caught in events and feelings beyond the human scale and beyond the power of human consciousness to alter?

I once read an article about the Titanic. Forget the movie. The essence of that catastrophe was that there were a hundred and some-odd human mistakes. Any one of them, had it been caught, would have prevented the disaster. But none were caught. I never used to believe in predestination. But there was no break in the chain of events and the "unsinkable" ship sank.

Like my mother. For that is where my dark spiral of thoughts begins and ends. In Mother's old age she fell prey to the dragon—the system—and whatever gods possessed her specific, individual "caretakers." Ultimately, the Gods of Greed and Corruption who rule the dragon claimed her life.

Jung says that outside the field of ego consciousness, a person has little awareness and consequently control of the complexes and archetypes that possess them. Is that what happened—will always happen? It's not just that her death was awful and unnecessary. What haunts me beyond the mini-cataclysm of her small, individual tragedy is the inescapable chronology of it.

Her cancer led to chemotherapy, which at one point included prednisone. Prednisone causes osteoporosis. When Mother fell in her yard years after the cancer, her prednisone-generated osteoporosis resulted in a broken hip. Her broken hip led to three hip operations. Mother went from her third hip operation into the nursing care system where, while my problems prevented me from protecting her, one instance of neglect or abuse after another killed her.

She could have skipped the last operation and gone straight to a wheelchair, but that was not in her character. Then was her death, *this* death, fated from the outset, inscribed on some cosmic calendar like an unvarying universal principle? Light travels at 93 million miles per second. Was her fate as irrevocable as a universal constant like the speed of light? If so, is that true for all of us, individually and collectively? Are we all, with our singular spirits and shared commonalities, compelled by the gods with our futures inked onto that glittering calendar with no option for changing the path or the date?

It is the end of April. My mother's been dead four months, and I'm still reeling, dazed and shell-shocked in the aftermath of the final half-year of her life. And it sometimes seems to me that my mother was claimed by a chain of events from which no diversion, no miraculous flight or further heroic transformation had ever been possible. And if indeed my mother's final six months were as inexorable as they seem, if her last road held no hope of reprieve, if nothing could have saved her, then the question that comes to me, of everything, is, what's the point?

I don't want to believe this. But it often seems to me there was no other way her life could have gone from the moment the first cancer cell took root in her body and one, two, three, the dominoes fell.

Redwood

Movement. I stand and look. Susie at last is slogging along toward me up the walkway. She's halfway past the house in front, approaching Mother's gate. She carries more cardboard boxes for those of my mother's things I will take home. I look at my watch. Fifteen minutes since she dropped me off. I must have died—my whole life has flashed before my eyes in that time.

"How far from here did you have to park?" I grab up my set of cardboard boxes from the rusted garden table as she reaches me. I walk a step ahead of her, over the high crests in the buckling walkway.

"Just down the street. I was afraid of the dogs."

"Dogs?" I remember some dogs running around. I'd ignored them.

"The pit bulls. They wouldn't let me out of my car. Finally, this guy came out of his house. I had to yell for help and he called them."

"I didn't realize they were pit bulls."

"That's why they didn't go after you. You weren't afraid."

Wild pit bulls and gangs. Good advertisement. Maybe I *can* keep the house.

We plod forward, she, blonde, and me, brunette, both of us wearing jeans and old sweatshirts; both, old gals in our fifties. But here at my mother's house, that's not my only self. As always happens here, the others are beginning to emerge. I am a child and a teen, a young woman and an older one, an orphan and my mother's daughter.

***

Hanging a little off its hinges, the screen door opens onto the three steps leading up to the redwood deck. Deep within myself I stall for an epoch before ascending these steps that will take me into the house that is as crowded with emotions and memories, old and recent, as it is with Mother's stuff.

I pull on the screen door. It resists, as recalcitrant as Mother herself sometimes proved. I drag it back. Somehow there is something of myself in its resistance as well.

It gives with a grudging squeal. I shove through with my boxes, Susie patient behind me.

Climbing the first step, I observe something on the redwood arch that frames the screen door. It draws my attention. Leaning toward it I see on the doorframe the shiny surface of the wood peeling away, revealing some pale old timber beneath. Until this very moment I've believed the deck was redwood. But I am noticing for the first time in my life that this doorframe is only painted to look like redwood. This must be true of the whole deck—a fact which disappoints me unduly, deepens my sadness yet further.

I glance up at the house, the bogus redwood walls, the rain-warped front door and, on either side of it, the wide windows. One faces out from the living room and the other, on the other side of the door, from the kitchen. I see again my mother puttering there around the stove and sink, as she did so often when I ascended these steps.

Abruptly, something surprising moves within me.

Last week I brought the first contractor into the house to give me an estimate on the work needed. He took one step inside and said, "It's like going back in time." I smiled at his whimsy.

Peering into the kitchen window now, I think about how, in my teens, Mother made me eat with her and I couldn't stop; and how, forty years later, Mother and I, from love, often shared a chicken. She cooked it; she had the oven, and I, only a burner. With each new chicken meal, I called to warn her, "It's bloody at the bone. You better cook it a little more before you eat it." Each time she ejaculated in bewilderment, "I've cooked and cooked it. I cooked it for hours. I don't know how this keeps happening!"

One day, along with the pile of newspaper clippings and health articles she sent me every week, a cartoon arrived. It showed a man with silverware in either hand. He is staring in bewilderment at the empty plate before him while, flying off through the air, is his dinner—the chicken.

My smile returns, my own whimsy.

It's like going back in time for me, too. Perhaps the long scale of memories I've allowed myself today have benefited me after all.

Reaching the deck, I feel my old selves stir. All our pasts, Mother's and mine, begin to emerge from the damp shadows before me. Once I'm inside the house, I will almost be able to smell the pasta and chicken and chili, and hear Mother's loud guffaws override the old accusations. Our various selves will take up life again inside my flesh. "Listen," I say to Susie. "I need to sit outside for a few more minutes. Do you mind?"

"Are you okay?" She casts an anxious glance at me.

"Yes." But I have no idea. "Why don't you make yourself some coffee? You don't have to start till I come in."

"No, it's okay. I'll start."

"Okay, thanks. I won't be too long."

Susie goes inside, closing the door behind her to keep in the warmth she will elicit from the furnace, if she remembers where the thermostat is. Well, I'll be in soon. I sink onto the lumpy rocking chair facing the house, with all Mother's junk around me on the deck I once thought of as redwood. I rock the half-inch this space allows and listen for the birds my mother loved. They don't sing in the heavy gray air. But still I listen. I listen for my mother.

"I love to learn," she always said. I remember how, as she went from one room to another, Mitch and I could easily lose her. Oh, the numerous times Mother was supposed to call me back from her bedroom with some note she'd gone after—a phone number, a product label, a clipping. Or I waited on the phone while she ambled to her living room desk to snatch a piece of paper to write down information I wanted to give her. But she didn't pick up the extension or call me back.

And then there were the times about which Mitch told me. My mother had trekked off to put laundry into the dryer or take it out and she didn't return to him, as she was supposed to do, any more than she'd gotten back to me. She'd disappeared. Again. But we didn't worry. For one could always count on finding her, on such occasions, paused midstream, her erstwhile task forgotten. A piece of reading matter had commandeered her attention and she'd stopped wherever she was, too fascinated to move, standing or in later years sitting down for two hours to read whatever it was.

Perhaps even now she stands in the service porch, laundry in one hand, a book or periodical in the other, or she has paused in the short narrow hallway of the old house, or she sits on the bed in the small spare bedroom, reading something that has caught her eye as she was on her way elsewhere.

Not all journeys back into the house consist of pain. In fact, the reverse. How could I have forgotten?

Found Treasures

In the dark of the Underworld treasures gleam, and I do not hesitate to plunder. On my very first day back at the house, I espied Mother's wonderful Mexican silver bracelet and plucked it from atop the vanity in her bedroom; I wear it today. And in a cracked, chipped, porcelain, antique Chinese jewelry box, I found the sterling silver pins she purchased in Mexico and always wore, and a few Matisse earrings. The Chinese box itself, while monetarily worthless, I also love.

Sometimes a wholly unexpected treasure appears. Prints, for instance, hang everywhere in the house. "What's this?" Susie said on our first expedition when we were nearly done for the day. "It's signed."

I glanced over. She stood before a framed etching that hung over the furnace. I'd always found that black and white picture intimidating. Inside a circle two muscular, half-clad men meet in hand-to-hand, closed-fist combat. The lines are strong, the testosterone overpowering.

I joined Susie for a closer look. She pointed. Astonished, I saw what I'd never seen in all the years of my life. Penciled in beneath the circle that enclosed the two men, the artist had inscribed neatly: "To Hortense With Love Fletcher Martin."

In that moment I began to appreciate and love the print. Suddenly a treasure, it also became an instant object of intrigue. When I got it home, I called a vendor I knew from the swap meets I explore. He checked e-Bay and called me back a few days later. "Fletcher Martin was a DWP artist, pretty well known, in the forties in San Francisco."

My mother lived in San Francisco in the forties. That's where she met my father. She never mentioned Fletcher Martin. And now here is this work of art from their relationship. Which was—? "With love." Friendship? Romance? What important story of hers have I missed, and what further riddles did Mother leave here among the artifacts of her life? She was not a secretive person. That's one of the things Mitch loved most about her. She was so open about everything that there were things she just never thought to mention. Her death has transformed them into eternal mysteries. Might I roust more of them from crevices or corners, herd them from cupboards and closets?

And of course with my new, larger apartment I can take home some of her furniture, a dresser, the armoire, her stereo, one of her metal file cabinets. But, if I find it, the greatest tangible treasure will be her book, the one she compiled from the humorous exchanges she excerpted from the trial transcripts she typed in her youth; the book whose name she took, in her classic love of clever word-play, from the popular Perry Mason television show. In that series the famous fictional attorney is wont to object to the judge, "That is incompetent, irrelevant and immaterial!" Mother entitled her book, *Incompetent, Irreverent and Immaterial!*

Mother, where is your book? Where did you put it? Or, where did I?

I do have the poem she wrote for me when I was a child. This single piece of her literary aspirations I've managed to rescue. In fact I look back to the moment she read it to me on the phone. Had I no curiosity? I cannot fathom how the moment slipped past. I was unsurprised by her talent but blown away by her skill. "This is fantastic!" I told her and never asked, "With that talent, why did you give up writing?" What could have stopped her? What happened to everything else she must have written? Now there is only the poem and her missing book.

Where is it? She gave me a copy twenty years ago. I immediately misplaced it. I always thought I'd get another from her. I never got around to asking. Where did she put the box that contained her copies? Did she hide it during a paranoid delusion? Did she know where it was but not think to tell me? Did she drop it down a *cenote?*

Did I toss it by accident?

Two weekends ago I began clearing out her bedroom four-drawer cabinet, pulling from it one health file after another and stuffing them into a garbage bag. I'd forgotten about her book and deliberately refused to focus on her scrupulously prepared file labels. They evoked too painful a picture of her: *She sits at her desk and, with the efficiency she learned in her office work and brought home, she categorizes and types the labels: "Diabetes," "Herbology," "Acupuncture," "Hoxy," "Gerson," "Donsbach Clinic."* I also have avoided thinking about how collecting these files had become her life's work, for neither Suzann nor I nor anyone else I know has room to keep them. And so I throw them out, one by one, my eyes closed on the labels.

Last Saturday morning I suddenly remembered my mother's book. But racing out to the trash bins, I found that the garbage truck had taken everything away since Susie's and my previous visit. Guilt burns a hole through my stomach. I was unable to find Mother's copies of her book anywhere in the house, though I looked furiously the rest of that day. But many files remain to be sorted. Perhaps among them I'll find it.

And there is one treasure, intangible, the greatest one, and never lost. The last time I visited Mother here, we stood in the service porch. I helped her fold the warm clothes she pulled from the dryer. Even warmer summer air poured in through the wide screen. We were once more discussing her upcoming operation. She again told me not to feel bad if she died. But this time she interjected something new into the conversation. She said, "No matter what happens, just remember that we loved each other. That's what counts."

***

Every time I come here, I resist entering the house, an impulse especially potent today. I don't want to feel that much pain. I have fled my pain in order to keep going: that is what I've told myself. First, to help my mother and now to get on with my own life, I've refused to visit my dark sister self, my mourning Erishkigal self. I've been afraid of losing my power to her.

But of course the reverse is true. The more I've pushed my pain aside, the more forcefully it has returned through panic attacks and an immobilizing sorrow. It is precisely my flight from the past that has given so much power to the Queen of the Dead. So today I have dared to let myself remember fully.

Just as I feared, I find myself possessed by Grief. But that is not the end of the story. Inanna does get back to the World of Light. Can I learn from her wisdom?

Before she descends, Inanna arranges with her servants to come and get her, to save her from her sister. And so after three days they come. They save her by sitting with Erishkigal, whose husband has died. They surround Erishkigal. They moan when she moans, they weep and scream when she does. They mirror her pain back to her, with compassion, until at last she is able to accept it.

Released from the grip of her eternal grief, Erishkigal, Goddess of the Underworld, releases her sister from the wall where she's hung her. Inanna returns to the World of Light from the World of the Dead. Symbolically, Inanna is reborn and her story represents the rebirth that comes from embracing your helpless grief.

I rock back and forth the little inch that my space here affords, in my lumpy rocking chair, back and forth, back and forth (like my mother in her last days). As my tears fall, I comfort myself as best I can, telling myself with compassion, *Yes, this is what happened, and it hurts, it hurts, it hurts.*

The Glow

I wipe the salty damp streaks from my eyes and cheeks. As I stand, I find my attention drawn back to the side of the wooden doorframe arching over the deck steps. With a frisson of hope, a nascent, irrational delight, I lean over to re-examine it. Careful of splinters, I run my fingers along the damp curl of wood where it peels back, polished and shiny on one side, splintery and dull on the other; the redwood that isn't redwood. But maybe, I re-evaluate, it is. What do I know? Maybe what peels back is not paint covering cheap wood but instead some varnish on actual redwood, a finish which makes the planks beneath it simply look paler by comparison. The pale rust flesh of real redwood.

When I was five or six, Mother remodeled the house, a bold move for a single woman. That's when the redwood deck went in. Somehow, now, to discover the redwood might be real brings unexpected light all through me and I remember something else.

Despite the current state of the house, both the listing, varmint-infested structure and the chaos inside, the banks of detritus from Susie's and my weekend salvaging here, despite it all, everyone I have taken inside—the contractor, estate salespeople, real estate agents, possible renters, a friend who'd never been here—all like the feel of the interior. They feel good here. They feel at home. For Mother's smile, that changed over the last quarter of a century from the placating version she must have learned in her childhood and that she tried to pound into me in mine—her smile, that changed with so much else about her—now casts a gentle glow within and around her house.

In the glow of that smile, it comes to me. You're here and then you're gone, and all that's left are the clues and traces of your passing: My mother's house, and the things in her house, and the ghost trails of the heart, the people she helped, the people she loved and who loved and remember her.

I won't be falsely positive. Her experience was terrible; and it could happen to me. Yet for this moment, regardless of my doubts, my grief, my daze and dumb shock, my often dark sense of fate, a little whisper or shimmer rises from within the void her death left in the world. Having cured herself of a fatal lymphoma, my mother inspired everyone she met and helped whoever asked. A quarter of a century after her cancer, with the strength of her will and a final flash of brilliance, she was eliminating the impairments in her brain. She was pulling her mind back from whatever abyss called to her, and although she collided with forces more powerful than any personal fate, a small personal triumph lingers in the air and bears her essence: her intelligence, laughter, generosity, imagination, fascination with life, and the glow of her unique spirit.

And all at once I recognize the obvious, and a kind of ecstasy elevates me. This agonizing Grief that I carry for my mother, which seems to extend infinitely in all directions of space and time; this Grief which, having once come to exist, has now always existed and always will—this Grief has a counterpart. That counterpart, equally transcending space and time, is Love. This is something I suddenly *know*.

***

I have somehow leapt into a completely new place. Though I creak and yank against my resistance, my fears, my precarious and insubstantial faith, I know with absolute conviction (even if only for a single moment) that, like Grief, Love is a non-local event and that every loving act and relationship lives, and has lived, forever.

Inevitably, it occurs to me that if personal love transcends the space-time continuum, then why not collective love? Every genuine act of compassion strengthens the non-local quantum vibration that enables the next compassionate act. Every step on the march toward wisdom and peace enables the next one to occur more easily everywhere. And if this is true, or only partially true, and we act on it, still we might change our collective fate.

Then a truly outlandish idea takes hold. Should we fail to save our Earth, our actions can still affect other sentient beings elsewhere in the universe. Our private and collective acts of love and peace can strengthen those quantum resonances universally and make it just a little easier for all beings everywhere and always to act with love, to save or enhance their own societies, environments, and interactions with each other and the other creatures in their lives.

Normally I despise sentimentality. In particular, heart-shaped icons and talk of angels put me in a diabetic coma. But now I smile, bemused if not giddy with this mythology that has come to me. (Am I ready to telemarket my own fuzzy-wuzzy airy-fairy LA cult?) I picture little angels of sympathetic vibration carrying messages of love and peace to extraterrestrial aliens on strange, new worlds...

I've been to the Underworld but I'm back, with an inkling of true inner peace. I've been to the Kingdom of the Dead and I'm reborn (even if not in every cell).

And then I think: if this picture of the universe contains any genuine insight, then here is another: the ability to outwit or disobey the gods is also an archetypal experience.

In the West the dragon has a negative character and symbolizes the "system." But in the East the dragon represents benevolent energy and power. There will always be dragons. But perhaps after all we can choose our dragon as we can choose other archetypes. The dragon can symbolize a *benevolent* system, one that supports individuals, families, communities and our common institutions. Each effort toward such a system strengthens that resonance, archetype, god: We can choose to summon a benevolent dragon who, with thunderously roaring wings, breathes the fire of creation and hope into the future of human (and alien) enterprise.

At any rate this is the dragon I invoke within myself, the dragon of a new benevolent psychological system. If I can just maintain it—or remember how to call it back when I falter.

***

How have I gotten here? By following the path I've followed all my life: searching for my "true self" after I myself have buried it, and then uncovering it again little by little. After denying my feelings, I've finally let them in, with a mirroring compassion. With empathy.

But already, even as I think this, my little bubble of cosmic glory is shrinking, my transcendent bliss lifting away. Ordinary reality collapses back around me, the damp morning, gray and cold; the quiet; the jacaranda tree; the purple blossoms; the redwood deck; the vacant house.

But one thing remains of my Inanna moment. I still know I can journey to the Underworld and not get stuck there forever. I can let myself relive Mother's and my relationship and feel the emotions more fully each time. I can embrace all of my mother's selves and all of mine. Nor, as I learned from my mother, do I have to be perfect in such emotional courage in order to find my own grace.

Meanwhile, my mother's inner glow still warms and lights the old house. Her smile inhabits and emanates from it. That is the truth that will prevail over this day and the next, and over the terrible images of what happened to her, images that will certainly continue to return to me at night for some time, with the tears I will finally let flow.

"Just remember," she said, "that we loved each other."

Yes, Mother, I tell her. *I remember.* Then I cross the furniture-gorged deck, turn the rattly knob of the rain-warped front door and push it open.

Once more I step inside my mother's house.

Epilogue

This was Susie's last trip with me to the house to clear it out. She could give up no more time. I couldn't do it alone and, as I expected, no one else could help me. I did return with a few other friends for odds and ends. Then I sold the house "as is."

The new owner found, among Mother's effects, her book, and gave it to me. A few weeks later, as I finished unpacking at my new apartment, I found the copy she gave me long ago.

The new owner of her house told me, with sensitivity, "Another family will be starting a new life in your mother's house."

***

If I recall correctly an interview I heard some years ago, a prominent physicist stated that the speed of light, contrary to what we've been told, is not a constant. It was assigned 93 million miles an hour for the sake of convenience but in fact it fluctuates, if only slightly.

Excerpt from.

INCOMPETENT, IRREVERENT AND IMMATERIAL!

Compiled by Hortense Gusick

Q: When you had taken your eyes off the traffic coming southbound and you looked to your right, you didn't change your body; it was just your head that you changed?

***

Q: What type was your prior accident?
A: It was a rear-end accident.
Q: Automobile?

***

Mr. Jones: Counsel, I want you to notice the ridges on the plaintiff's teeth.
Mr. Thomas: I can see nothing. However, I am not a dentist, and at the time of trial the teeth will speak for themselves.

***

Q: You were in the room when the doctor examined your husband, you say. Did you see him hit his knee with that little rubber hammer?
A: Yes.
Q: Did he look into his eyes, feel his neck, tap his chest?
A: Yes.
Q: Did he pull his chart?
A: I beg your pardon?

EATING MARCH

by Hortense Gusick

(To be spoken on a children's record, by one narrator or in choral verse, or used as verse with music)

Oh, food is delicious
And eating is fun!

When Mommy calls me
I come at a run!

Run to the table
As fast as I'm able

And eat!
Eat!
Eat a bite of beet!

Drink!
Drink!
Drink milk that's smooth as silk!

Chew!
Chew!
I chew good and so do you!
Chew green pepper and carrot and beans and potatoes
And liver and lettuce and round red tomatoes

And laugh!
Laugh!
How I laugh and I chatter
As I clean up my platter!

Then say,

"H E Y !
I'M THROUGH!
ARE YOU?"

About the Author

At age ten Alexa Wolf won first place for her age group in a poetry contest sponsored by the International Women's League for Peace and Freedom. Ten years later she won a fellowship to the MacDowell Colony. Her published work includes stories for the *LA WEEKLY* including a cover story, *THE NEW YORK NATIVE* and an article for the C. G. Jung Institute journal, *PSYCHOLOGICAL PERSPECTIVES.* When misdiagnosed for HIV/AIDS, she appeared on numerous television and radio programs including THE TODAY SHOW, a Dan Rather special and OPRAH!

Alexa lives in Los Angeles. She wrote most of this book in the company of her little bird, Captain Kirk the Parakeet.

www.AlexaWolfOnline.com

Please feel free to contact Alexa at
alexawolf@AlexaWolfOnline.com
She welcomes all comments and questions.

Made in the USA
Middletown, DE
13 November 2026

36932802R00245